DOCTOR INTEGRALIST'S
PRESCRIPTION TO
HEALTHY
LIVING

DR. BIPRAJIT PARBAT

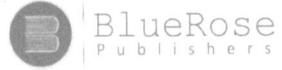

© **Dr. Biprajit Parbat 2021**

All rights reserved

All rights reserved by author. No part of this publication may be reproduced, stored in a retrieval system or transmitted in any form or by any means, electronic, mechanical, photocopying, recording or otherwise, without the prior permission of the author.

Although every precaution has been taken to verify the accuracy of the information contained herein, the author and publisher assume no responsibility for any errors or omissions. No liability is assumed for damages that may result from the use of information contained within.

First Published in April 2021

ISBN: 978-93-5427-545-6

BLUEROSE PUBLISHERS
www.bluerosepublishers.com
info@bluerosepublishers.com
+91 8882 898 898

Cover Design:
Nirmal

Typographic Design:
Deepika Matpal

Distributed by: BlueRose, Amazon, Flipkart

Dedication

The book is dedicated to my beloved parents, wife and children.

Acknowledgment

I am really thankful to my mother who always inspires me to go the extra miles in my life. My father is a silent contributor to my success, and I pay my gratitude to him. My beloved wife and my daughter, whose patience and silent companionship help me to make research and write, sometimes really astonish me. I owe my thanks to all the researchers whose researches have enriched my writing (I have mentioned their works in the reference sections of the book). Without their hard work the book would not be here today. I extend my gratitude to all.

Preface

I do believe in a 360-degree integral approach as disease prevention is necessary for high performance and happiness in life. The approach is equally important for physical and mental health that helps people to fit his natural evolution with his modern-day life. There are personal and professional factors which affect your overall heath. Our choice of food, our scope and requirement of exercise, our scope of sleep, and our requirements of stress management are determined by both our personal and professional factors. Personal factors are your– daily routine, taste preferences for food, habits, beliefs and focus. Professional factors are– work schedule, type of job, place and movement needed for the job. The inclusive and integrative approach to transform lives will save humanity from diseases, disabilities and death by millions. In this integral approach lay the four pillars of health that should be actualized for the purpose: FOOD, EXERCISE, SLEEP and STRESS MANAGEMENT. A common-sized overall guidance, for all those who are aiming towards healthy living, has been provided. It has its inherent flaws, one being that it is not customized to someone's personal and professional factors. That's where you will need professional help. But I believe many of you will be benefitted by just following the simple advice for healthy living. That's where this book comes in.

You can read more about the related topics on my website – biprajitparbat.com

Content

Introduction 1

Our Natural Food & Eating Window 12

    The BIG problem with our food habits - 15

    A short story from our daily life: 18

    The science behind the story: 19

    Victor Considers: 20

    The solution: 21

    The science behind the solution: 22

    The eating window – 23

    Quick Tip: 24

    Benefits: 25

    Table 01 Organic Sources of Essential Nutrients 30

    Table No. 02 Organic Sources of Vitamins 32

    Table 03 Organic Sources of Minerals 35

    References: 37

Exercise-The minimum maintenance work for our body 40

    "Exercise is a celebration of what your body can do. 40

    Not a punishment for what you ate" 40

    Anonymous 40

    The ordinary benefits of aerobic exercises are as follows: 41

The beliefs that need to be changed: 42

Exercise Intensity: 44

Timing for Exercise: 45

Exercise Type: 46

The solution: 47

The science behind the solution: 48

Quick tips: 48

Move your sub-conscious and stop procrastinating – 49

Recognition: 50

Declaration: 50

Practise meditation and mindfulness to overcome the procrastination towards exercise. 50

References: 52

Recovery and Sleep 54

"Life is not merely being alive, but being well." 54

Wrong beliefs about our sleep 54

The little science of circadian rhythm 56

A short story from our daily life: 57

The science behind the story: 58

The solution: 60

The science behind the solution: 60

Quick tips: 62

More discussion on physical exercise can be found in the next chapter. 64

Take care of your sleep – 64

Journaling 65

References: 65

Why stress management is important? 68

The following 10 changes happen in our body following long-standing stress: 69

Why long-term stress is bad for our health 70

How an emergency quick response "stress" can create cascades of long-standing problems in the human being? 73

The Little Biology to Understand Stress 75

Part I: Psycho-neurology – 75

The subconscious mind – 75

Chemical brain- 81

The responsive CEO, the reactive CEO & the executive – 85

Our mind is like an Operating System 87

The upgrade needs:- 88

The process to upgrade: 90

The science behind it – 90

Move Into "The Zone Of Execution" - Usc The Secrets Of Sports Psychology 92

Why Can't We Do Things Even If We Want To Do Them Consciously? 93

What Should We Do To Improve Our Execution? .. 95

Failure to execute at will is a very big source of stress and anxiety. So, let us discuss few ways to improve execution: 96

Make stress your friend and ride it like a SPORTS CAR. 101

   Where is the "BRAKE?" Why it is NOT working? 104

   Journaling – 104

   Practice Stillness Of Non-judgmental Awareness– SNA Meditation.. 104

   Write down the following benefits of SNA in your journal- 109

The S.T.O.P. 111

(Self-talk Optimizer Protocol) 111

   "Don't be a VICTIM of the negative talk, remember. 111

   YOU are listening." – Bob Proctor 111

   The short story 112

   The Story Ends- What has happened? 114

   There are more examples 116

   So, what would be the solution? 117

Flexibility is the KEY 119

   R.P.M. World Point of View- (Relative, Probabilistic and Multifactorial)........................... 119

   Power of Query- 121

   Install the art inside your sub-conscious- 124

- Rule The Reactions 126
  - "Between stimulus & response, there is a space. In that space is our power to choose our response. In our response lies our growth & our freedom." 126
  - Why is it essential to install the space? 128
  - Become the CONFIDENT and SECURE SELF ... 129
  - Install the space and rule the reactions – 130
- Mind Your Productive Categories 132
  - "Productivity" 132
  - The science behind productive thoughts– 135
  - Manage Your FOCUS 136
  - Focus is a very useful but finite currency. Spend with care. 136
  - Know Your "Step 1" 138
  - Manage Your FOCUS 140
  - What to do? 143
- Transform With the Muscle of Gratitude 144
  - "Gratitude is a vaccine, an antitoxin, and an antiseptic." ~ John Henry Jowett, 1863 – 1923 144
  - WHAT IS GRATITUDE? 144
  - HOW TO FEEL GRATITUDE? 145
  - STUDIES AND RESEARCH 149
  - HOW GRATITUDE INFLUENCES PHYSICAL HEALTH? 151

HOW DOES GRATITUDE INFLUENCE
MENTAL HEALTH? 153

Gratitude also affects our work. Here are
some incredible statistics about the influence
of gratitude at the workplace: 154

Expression of gratitude – 156

Minimalism 158

Problems of so many choices and so much
information - 158

Reframe concept of minimalism – 162

Bring the Pareto principle in your life – 163

Minimalism decision matrix 163

Managing things with minimalism 164

Own the power of "Impermanence" & "Time." 166

References: 168

Introduction

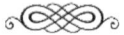

Integrative medicine is oriented to healing, which takes into account the whole person (body, mind and spirit). It encompasses conventional and natural medicine, making available to the patient all possible instruments for healing. With integrative medicine, people can be masters of their health, and the role of an integrative doctor is to guide and accompany them throughout the healing process. Furthermore, stress, in its four varieties (chemical, physical, emotional and spiritual), is a factor that must be learned to combat in order to prevent disease and seek longevity.

The profile of healthcare is rapidly changing. Various trends over the past decades, both in the world of conventional medicine and beyond, are changing the nature of healthcare and the context in which physicians' practice. Total drug spending is increasing at an alarming rate. We have a better understanding, now, of the magnitude of the problems associated with adverse drug reactions and associated deaths. In the meantime, the consumer movement, fuelled by access to the health information on the internet, has led to a dramatic increase in interest in alternative and complementary medicine. The public spends considerable sums of money, out of their own pockets, on this integrative approach.

Another disturbing trend is the rise in people suffering from obesity, and the resulting complications for the past decade or so. It validates the fact that today the biggest threats to health cannot be effectively cured merely with medication or surgery. Many of the problems encountered in primary care include social, spiritual, and lifestyle factors. Talking about the provider side of the situation, professional dissatisfaction and physical stress are now recognized as crucial issues that must be addressed in order to be able to provide optimal care.

In the present times, physicians are responding in various ways to these changes in their work environment. Some people reassess their priorities and try to achieve a better balance in their personal lives. Others are trained in alternative interventions and offer these services to their patients. Still others are developing their skills in lifestyle and wellness counselling and health promotion. At present, however, these changes are optional and inconsistently implemented, and medical education has not consistently adhered to them.

A new movement in healthcare has incorporated these disparate trends and sought to formally articulate a new vision for medicine- a vision that responds to the problems we are currently facing and attempts to address them. This movement is commonly referred to as "integrative medicine." The first textbooks have already been written, and a consortium of medical schools has been established to transform the undergraduate education curricula to reflect the vision of this approach. But what exactly is "integrative medicine?" As mentioned above, it is the healing medicine that takes into account the whole person (body, mind and soul). This includes all the aspects of a person's way of life. It focuses on the therapeutic relationship as well as uses all appropriate therapies, both alternative and conventional.

Contrary to popular belief, "integrative" is not only a philosophy of the care of patients but also a description of a specific array of practices. This approach emphasizes the prevention of diseases with a focus on enhancing the benefits of lifestyle and nutrition interventions. This approach is entirely inclusive of the medical therapy that is based on guidelines. Moreover, integrative cardiology aims to empower patients as much as possible with therapeutic plans and health goals that are developed collaboratively.

Integrative cardiology is increasingly important as it addresses all the unmet needs in the conventional approach to medicine. Despite the rapid technological advances in the field of medicine, the US Centres for Disease Control and Prevention (CDC) released a report that describes the recent decline in cardiovascular diseases that are basically a manifestation of problems related to the lifestyle such as diabetes and obesity.

Lifestyle and nutrition are not given proper attention during the practice of cardiology. This means that there is no mention of the importance of lifestyle and nutrition in the training of this disease. **An integrative approach of cardiology seeks to correct this deficiency by emphasizing lifestyle and nutrition as integral parts of the overall therapeutic plan.**

Adoption of this integrative cardiology approach is also a good idea because it can result in improved outcomes over time. For instance, implementation of lifestyle modifications or atrial fibrillation after an ablation procedure can do wonders for a person's recovery.

Associated Treatment Modalities

1. Nutrition

It is an indisputable fact that nutrition is an important aspect of medical care. The diet of an individual is crucial in the integrative cardiology mode. It has been found that nutritional interventions are the cornerstone of cardiac care for the treatment and prevention of cardiovascular disease.

2. Mind/Body Therapy

Research suggests that there is a strong connection between a person's emotional state and cardiovascular thought. An individual's thoughts and state of mind play a significant role in the health of their heart. This integrative approach focuses on the connection between the mind and the body. Medication and cognitive behavioural therapy are more traditional approaches, and the integrative model that can be taken to treat cardiovascular diseases includes breathing exercises, meditation, healing touch, yoga, Reiki, and biofeedback.

3. Mind/Heart Connection

Takotsubo syndrome is perhaps the best example of how the mind and the heart are closely connected. This condition refers to a severe and acute failure of the left ventricle, which is increased due to psychological stress. The Takotsubo syndrome is the perfect example of the manifestations of emotional state and stress in the cardiac health of a person.

4. Meditation

Studies suggest that the mind-heart connection can be harnessed to prevent ischemic heart disease. A controlled study, conducted on meditation, reported that the people who meditated experienced a staggering 48% lower risk of strokes and all-cause mortality. Although the underlying mechanism remains unclear, it was discovered that meditation favours blood pressure. Stress reduction, which is based on mindfulness, is also associated with an attenuated inflammatory response.

5. Healing Touch

Most health professionals are unfamiliar with the approach of the healing touch. Healing touch and Reiki have become quite popular modalities in recent times. They are used for both pain reduction and stress management. In both these approaches, practitioners use hand motions and a light touch on the body in order to redirect energy. Irrespective of the mechanism, several patients have reported experiencing substantial relief over the years. In a recent study, conducted on 237 inpatients who were recovering from coronary bypass surgery, patients who received the healing touch performed better with lower anxiety scores. Moreover, their hospital stats were reduced significantly as opposed to the other patients who were not subjected to the therapy.

6. Environment

Another thing that influences cardiovascular disease-related risk factors is the physical environment. In a study, researchers monitored the ambulatory heart rate of individuals in urban settings. This was monitored with and without the presence of greenery. People who regularly walked in urban green spaces had a lower ambulatory heart rate than those who lived in urban areas without the presence of much or any greenery. In this regard, a lower ambulatory heart rate in green spaces and parks reflects "biophilia," which is the innate affinity of people in regular contact with nature and the physical environment.

We need integrative approach to prevent diseases and their complications.

"Integrative medicine" is a medical practice that is concerned with offering a treatment that treats not just the disease but rather the patient as a whole. The relationship between a doctor and a patient is extremely important for integrative medicine since all treatment is based on the patient's individuality, taking into account aspects such as his/her personality and the way of relating to the world, among others.

Whether you want to prevent disease or prevent the complications of disease, you need to upgrade your lifestyle that has originally caused the disease.

The direct cost of prevention is way cheaper than the treatment of disease and its complications, even if I do not consider the loss of productivity in your career and business that is incurred when you have the disease and afterwards.

The act of prevention needs an integral approach that involves a 360-degree assessment and improvement of the lifestyle of a person. It helps him to fit his million-year-old natural evolution to the modern life style.

The holistic approach brings out the best productive and creative self.

One-dimension approach like only healthy eating or only exercising is not enough in today's world. A complete lifestyle transformation is necessary to cope with the fast-changing world. We are modifying our world at a very fast pace, yet our evolution remains almost same as the way it was a hundred years back. This is spawning stress and diseases, out of which almost 70% of them are lifestyle related. Food, exercise, sleep, daily routine, stress management and optimization are necessary to take the ownership of best productive and creative self.

Food is not something which we use fill up our stomach. Food is something our body uses to supply necessary ingredients towards the building of our body. We become the food we intake.

Our muscles needs minimum maintenance otherwise they will become weak. If our muscles become weak, our joints become weak too, as our joints are supported by our muscles. Exercise for minimum maintenance is necessary. Apart from that, exercise improves mood, motivation, blood circulation, metabolism – to name only a few.

Again, sleep is the most important part of living a healthy life. Our body regenerates daily at night when we sleep. It prepares itself to deal with the stress of the next day. Without proper sleep the body and brain suffer from daily regeneration. Long-term sleep deprivation is surely makes a way for the diseases and disabilities in future.

The fast-changing world is producing more stress than ever. We need physical and mental health strategies to manage the stress as we march forward. We should seek to keep the strength of our natural evolution by our side. Otherwise we will permit our lifestyle to give rise to physical and mental diseases. These can rob us of our productivity, creativity and happiness. Having a strategy in place is the need of the hour.

HeIt is believed that mediation should be an integral part of our regular life to maintain mental hygiene. A stress coping strategy should be in place for everyone to cope with the ever-changing world.

A 360-degree integral approach is necessary.

There are personal and professional factors which affect your overall heath. Your choice of food, your scope and requirement of exercise, your scope of sleep and your requirements of stress management are determined by both your personal and professional factors.

Personal factors are your - daily routine, taste preferences for food, habits, beliefs and focus.

Professional factors are – work schedule, type of job, place and movement required for the job.

Apart from the personal life, a person's profession controls more than one third of his daily activity and timing. Sometimes the timing of the office may be at night, sometimes the work pressure is at its peak and sometimes the job involves a lot of travelling. At times it requires you to sit for hours on your chair and while at other times it has the constant stress of talking, negotiating, rejecting, and so on.

Our job controls a significant part of our life style and contributes a significant amount to the physical and mental stress. Many a time people take the help of addictions as a part of their coping mechanism. This is not sustainable, as far their health is concerned.

A 360-degree integral approach means complete assessment of one's personal and professional requirement for the care of physical and mental health. Then a health strategy is formulated such

that it helps people to cope best with their personal and professional demand in natural way. Evidence-based scientific and medical knowledge is used to formulate the strategy. Then the person will be trained and given step-by-step guidance to apply the same. It takes about 3 to 6 months to become trained and accustomed to the new and upgraded lifestyle. The person will become physically fit, mentally resilient, more productive, happy and creative. It is a journey to become your best self physically and mentally in your own way. Prevention of disease and their complications would require such an integral approach.

There are scientifically proven techniques to prevent lifestyle-related physical and mental diseases. Now you can live a "good healthy life" by strengthening the four pillars of healthy life with "GOOD LIFE GOALS:" "FOOD, EXERCISE, SLEEP and STRESS MANAGEMENT." Live a healthy life with a healthy heart. These are hours of knowledge that no doctor has time to hand over to their patients. Thanks to digital media, I will be able to deliver these to you through this platform.

Our civilization has progressed more rapidly in the last 50 years than in the previous 250 million years of human history. The progress is changing our lives more quickly than ever. We have lit our nights with bright lights, information is pouring like rain in our lives, choices and processing of food are of infinite varieties and we move significantly less at work.

A newspaper had published a piece of news once: "A billionaire has been eaten by his own pet LION !!!" How is that even possible? A billionaire bought a baby lion and kept it inside a cage. He petted it well and loved it very much. He had started on a few projects and that made him very busy. One night he came home, drank a few pegs of whiskey before going to pay a visit to his baby lion. He opened the cage, and was attacked by an adult lion. The attack killed him instantly.

"It was for the last 3 years that he did not visit the house as he was very busy," the attendant started crying as he told this to the police officer-in-charge.

The police officer told, "Busy businessman, indeed. Never knew when his own lion got bigger than his lap!!!"

We, humans, are so busy building new things that we do not notice how much our habitat and habits have significantly changed over the last few decades. We can easily do things that are unnatural to our million years old human evolution. And these changes are not under our control. That is reality. We need to change our habits to match our modern civilization naturally with our natural evolution.

In simple words, I am asking you to learn about your body's needs. I believe with a little effort you can arrange your modern-day life in a way that fits with your million years old evolution.

In this journey of knowledge and realization I found the four pillars of our good health: "FOOD," "EXERCISE," "SLEEP" and "STRESS MANAGEMENT."

These are the suggestions that no physician is able to give to his patients due to lack of time. I am writing this book on general well-being to deliver to you the hours of knowledge which you would need to live life healthy.

These are the pillars that hold the vessel of a "GOOD LIFE." And no matter what goals we want to achieve in our life, we should have "**the four pillars of GOOD LIFE GOALS**" to begin with. Here is a prescription from a doctor, written in simple words, for leading a healthy life.

Our Natural Food & Eating Window

"Let food be thy medicine and Medicine be thy food." Hippocrates, 460 BC.

Our food is not something that we use to fill our stomachs. These are the supply system or ingredients that our body uses to regenerate almost all our body parts daily. The concept is that "we become our food" over a period of time. Our body and brain regenerate daily, especially when we sleep ("slow-wave sleep"), under the guidance of our growth hormones and by using the food components. The lack of essential nutrients reduces our body's process of regeneration and healing. We should become aware of whether we are supplying our body with proper nutrients; otherwise, our body's hunger signal will always remain "ON." Thus our desire to eat will remain making us eat more and more, and finally we will need apps and weighing machine to know how much food we should eat. Under this stress, where proper nutrients are constantly supplied at a reduced rate, our body will store more fat (more belly fat – more intra-abdominal and visceral fat). These lead to obesity and its complications.

Our body also has a hormonal system that can store food by using insulin and can handle stress by cortisol and adrenaline. We can regenerate using growth hormones while sleeping in an empty stomach. Both can't happen simultaneously. If we collect proper food for 12 hours, we should provide a decent 12 hours of regeneration window at night, with adequate sleep, so that our body can regenerate. This is now evidence-based science. With a time-restricted diet, your cholesterol level and insulin sensitivity improves. It restores your circadian rhythm (the necessary rhythm of hormones and homeostasis that changes in our body every 24 hours). Your hunger and satiety centres signal you so that you understand the requirement of food. You know when to eat and how much to eat. The sensitivity of these centres' functionality also improves. There is no need for an app and weighing machine to track your food intake.

But due to the regular marketing done by many food companies for processed and deep fried food, we consider those items as food. We also believe that refined and fried food counters as a source of food for us because of its easy availability and visibility. These are all food-like items – they smell like food and look like food. But without the essential nutrients which are spoiled during processing and frying, these are not considered as food anymore. Refined sugar causes more undulation of blood sugar & insulin; thus, we feel drowsy after an hour of taking such foods. Refined sugar is more harmful than the saturated fat itself. These foods cause more stress daily than any life events that we may have.

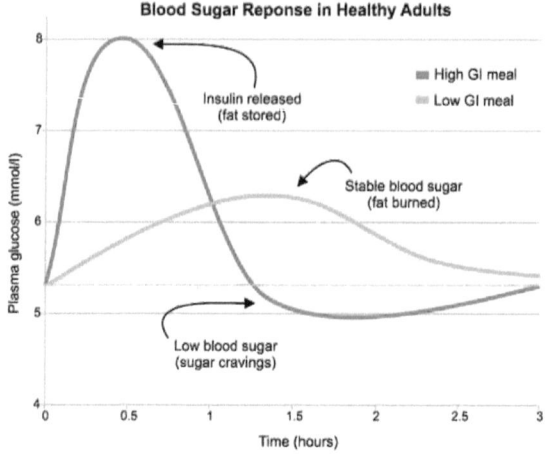

Figure 01: As you can see in the graph, the X-axis denotes time and it is denoted by 1/2hour, 1 hour, 1.5 hours, 2 hours, 2.5 hours like that. And in the Y-axis you can see plasma glucose level that is in the millimoles per litre scale.

The Glycemic Index (GI) is a relative ranking of carbohydrate in foods according to how they affect blood glucose levels. Carbohydrates with a low GI value (55 or less) are more slowly digested, absorbed and metabolized and cause a lower and slower rise in blood glucose and therefore usually in insulin levels.

The BIG problem with our food habits -

"Healthy eating" in recent times can be considered a myth. Every day people are struggling with their schedule to manage their personal and professional life. In the pursuit of doing so, "healthy eating" and leading an "active lifestyle" seem to be the two most impossible and unattainable tasks. Consequently, unhealthy eating and leading a sedentary lifestyle has resulted in an increased prevalence of chronic illnesses such as obesity, diabetes and cardiovascular diseases. International Diabetes Federation states that the incidence of diabetes within India's urban region ranges between 10.9% and 14.2% and that in rural India is between 3.0% and 7.8%. ICMR-INDIAB suggests that the prevalence of obesity in the Indian population is between 11.8% and 31.3% in men and 16.9% and 36.3% in women. Abdominal obesity is one of the primary risk factors that contribute to cardiovascular diseases and associated comorbidities. The prevalence of cardiovascular disorders in India has been estimated to be equivalent to 54.5 million. One in every four deaths, that takes place in India, is due to cardiovascular complications. Strokes and heart attacks, arising out of cardiovascular disorders, are causing more than 80% of the deaths. Research shows that premature mortality due to cardiovascular diseases has increased by 59%, from 23.2 million (in 1990) to 37 million, as documented in 2010. It is worth noting that integrating the two factors "healthy eating" and "leading an active lifestyle" can lead to a healthy and disease-free life.

- At first, before any change happens, we must acknowledge that we have been doing something wrong. We must admit that those wrong things come from the false beliefs which prevent us from doing activities need to be carried out. Some of those beliefs that you may consider changing are given here.

- We need to change
- We will discuss the few of our beliefs that are not serving us well.

Dieting means suffering – no, that's not right. The more natural food you take, the more energetic you will feel. The natural foods are tastier and soothing than the unnatural food-like substances. These food-like substances are mostly devoid of any particular essential nutrients in it (white rice, maida, refined sugar, all fried foods and equivalents – these are all damaged and processed food).

I do not have time for dieting – If you are taking food, you can always change the food you eat and the time window of eating.

Counting your calories is a must – Correct the types of food you eat and the eating window. The signalling problem that your body has lost about how much to eat and when you need to eat will be so well-functioning that you will not need any "weighing machine" or "calorie counting app" to measure your food. Your stomach and brain has more sophisticated machinery installed in them already. Just do not make them malfunction by eating refined or fried food and not eating for more than 8 to 12 hours a day.

Appetite suppression is a must – No, you do not need to suppress your hunger. Your appetite swing happens unnaturally because of the spoiled and processed food that you throw into your stomach at regular intervals. If you correct your choice of food and the eating window, you will never need to suppress your appetite and tolerate hunger.

* Fasting is bad for health – No, it is not. Science has proven that time-restricted food intake and prolonged night-time fasting, for at least 12 hours a day, are very beneficial for our health.

Re-framing older beliefs

Older beliefs –
Which are not serving the purpose of your health.

1. Food we take is to fill up the stomach and when we are hungry we can fill it up by anything.
2. Which tastes good & smell good are good food.
3. Fasting is bad for health.
4. All fats are bad and should be avoided.
5. We need to count our calories for healthy eating – as a guidance to how much to eat.

Newer beliefs –
which serves the Purpose of our health better.

1. Food is the necessary supply of ingredients for our health & immunity.
2. These may be FOOD-LIKE items with only calories and no essentials attached with it.
3. 12- 14 hours of fasting is good for health. Even doing exercise in the morning while fasting is good for health.
4. Fats are not that BAD. Only trans-fats are bad. Omega 3 fats are essential for our good health.
5. Correct your supply of nutrition and do NOT eat more than 12 hours a day. Your body's sensory system will guide you in a far more efficient way.

Figure 02: The left side shows the common older beliefs about food, those that are not serving our physical health well, and the right side shows the common newer beliefs, those that will serve our health in a far better way.

*All fats are bad – No, absolutely not. Our cell membranes are made up of cholesterol. We need the essential fatty acids for the proper functioning of our body and its hormones. It also helps us to absorb fat-soluble vitamins. Only processed and trans-fats are bad. Even grass-fed animal fats are good for our health.

Eating small meals frequently is better – If your hunger and satiety centres are functioning and you have a proper choice of natural food and feeding window – you will never need frequent and small meals. You will never need more than three meals a day. You will feel more satisfied and full with just two healthy meals per day.

** I can only request you to change these beliefs, if you have any. Own the natural human diet. Get rid of processed and fried foods. Correct your window of eating. That's all you need for a healthy food habit and thus a healthy body.

A short story from our daily life:

Victor is a 28-yearold man who works as a senior software manager in the 'XYZ' organization. Victor is based in another city, far from his hometown. He stays alone in a rented 1 BHK and manages to visit home only once a year. Victor's designation demands excessive workload and stringent monitoring of his subordinates. He leaves for his office every morning at 9 am. He munches on leftovers, from the night before, for breakfast. He hardly gets enough time from his schedule for a proper lunch and typically orders in a "cheese sandwich" or a "pizza." He leaves the office, exhausted, around 8 pm and relies on "takeaway meals" for dinner. He generally goes clubbing on the weekends with his mates and consumes excess alcohol. Victor consumes six to seven cups of coffee every day and smokes ten cigarettes each day. Fifteen months ago, when Victor joined the organization, he weighed 60kgs and his height was 5ft 7". Victor currently weighs 95 kgs and has been diagnosed with Class 1 Obesity. He finds it difficult to climb the stairs to reach his flat on the second floor. He feels sluggish, tired and experiences shortness of breath.

He has recently been experiencing chest pain and borderline blood sugar. The general physician has asked him to get specific tests done and suspects an underlying cardiovascular disease.

The reason behind narrating Victor's case is to explain the adverse impact of unhealthy eating and leading a sedentary lifestyle. It can be inferred from Victor's case that he spends almost 10 hours in his office where his body is stationary. He relies excessively on "takeaway meals" and convenient foods such as white bread and pizza. These food items are processed and are highly refined. They are devoid of essential nutrient value such as vitamins, minerals, protein or fibre. Also, Victor consumes excessive amounts of coffee that is rich in its sugar content and is unhealthy for the body. Victor smokes around ten cigarettes a day and drinks alcohol excessively on the weekends, which can be considered as the primary contributor to the present condition of his physical health.

> "The food you eat can be either the safest
> and most powerful form of medicine or
> the slowest form of poison."
>
> -Ann Wigmore.

The science behind the story:

On carefully analyzing Victor's case, the principles and scientific research findings can help us understand how the identified factors have resulted in Victor's current health condition. A research conducted by the Texas Heart Institution has shown that sedentary behaviour and obesity mutually co-exist and this kind of behaviour is the primary contributor to obesity. So, due to a lack of physical activity in his everyday routine, Victor was susceptible to obesity. Research further shows that excessive consumption of sugary fluid results in the excess intake of calories. The human brain is unable to register the calorie percentage and so the cumulative calorie intake increases. Excess consumption of sugar drives insulin resistance. It is linked to chronic illnesses such as Type II diabetes, cardiovascular disorders and non-fatty liver disease. The refined flour used in the making of pizza is devoid of the essential nutrient value. It increases cholesterol level, which, if unchecked, leads to blockage of blood vessels due to cholesterol deposition. The overall energy content of alcohol can be considered to be equivalent to the extra calories that increase the day's total calorie intake. The impact has been studied to promote over-eating, accompanied by the consumption of a high-fat diet, which results in excessive weight gain. Research studies also suggest that excessive smoking is associated with diabetes, metabolic syndrome, and an enhanced risk of cardiovascular disorders. Therefore excessive smoking can be linked to poor health outcomes, in the case of Victor.

Victor Considers:

Victor calls up his best friend, Samuel, and tells him about his present health condition. Samuel suggests Victor should take some steps to lose weight, to cure his obesity, and asks him to join the gym and follow a "keto diet." Victor's colleague, Sophia, browses the internet and suggests him to go on a "vegan diet" and join yoga classes. Victor's sister, Melanie, suggests that he should take supplements and go for rigorous weight loss training. Confused with so many advises, Victor starts smoking more, and is clueless about what to do.

The solution:

While Victor's well-wishers recommend him the most popular weight loss routine and diets, most of the information is half-baked and is not supported with evidence. Going for rigorous physical training or joining the gym would be extremely tedious for Victor as, at present, he finds it extremely tiring to climb the stairs of his apartment. Hence, this option does not seem feasible. The keto diet is associated with nutritional deficiencies, kidney damage and other health issues such as dehydration, constipation and fatigue. Therefore, complying with the keto diet is also not a feasible option for Victor. The vegan diet is associated with the consumption of only plant-based products. Studies prove that it can facilitate weight loss and reduce risks related to diabetes Type II and premature death. However, the diet's consumption deprives the body of nutrients such as Vitamin D, Vitamin B12, calcium, Omega-3 fatty acids, iron and zinc. This type of diet results in poor health outcomes.

Victor could not understand any of the mumbo-jumbo of so-called "dieting." He also failed to keep track of his daily calories through an app and with a weighing machine. What he could do was follow a simple lifestyle that would be feasible to him. So he did his research and started a possible lifestyle change towards mindful and healthy eating. **He gradually started removing all processed and fried food from his daily choice of food. He started eating more vegetables with some brown rice and at times he also ate oats. His body received essential fatty and amino** acids from eggs, fishes, peanuts, almonds and walnuts. His diet included one or two fruits per day; he restricted his coffee within three cups and stopped taking coffee after 3 pm. He slept soundly for seven to eight hours each night. He restricted his feeding window to 10 to 12 hours daily. He started the consumption of a balanced and proportionate diet that was rich in nutrient value. He added some light exercise, for around 10 minutes in the mornings, and began walking for 15 minutes, in the evenings, per day. He also does not drink more than two pegs of alcohol twice a week and gradually stopped smoking. That's all he did, and within four months of changing his lifestyle, the condition of his health improved a lot. Now he has become an average individual with a healthy lifestyle.

The science behind the solution:

Victor supplied his body with proper nutrition through whole food, fruits and vegetables with a high level of fibres. He ate food which was rich in essential amino acids and essential fatty acids. He also did not eat for more than 12 hours a day. His growth hormone action was enhanced and the fluctuations in blood sugar were reduced. Insulin sensitivity improved, as well. The body's healing rate was better as the essential amino acids, essential fatty acids, essential vitamins and minerals are present in higher quantities in unprocessed and natural foods. His hunger and satiety centres started functioning correctly. He does not feel hungry all the time now. He did not need to track his food by weighing machines and online applications. His own body became his guide to his eating habits.

The eating window –

2.5 million years ago, before the discovery of light, humans were majorly farmers, hunters and gatherers. They would have their first meal at around 6 to 8 am and their last meal at about 5 to 8 pm. The eating window back then would be of 8 to 12 hours, and their diet majorly comprised of high-fibre vegetables, whole grain foods and meat. These foods are enriched with phytochemicals, vitamins, minerals, essential fatty acids and essential amino acids, all of them being essential nutrients for the body. The fasting at night used to be for at least 12 hours. This food intake pattern facilitated improved digestion and improved action of the growth hormones (GH) that is responsible for the regeneration of our body while we sleep soundly. Research shows that the GH level is highest around midnight, and the hormone can work efficiently when the body is in its resting phase. That's why our forefathers led healthier lives with much lesser chronic lifestyle disorders such as obesity, diabetes, or cholesterol problems.

The key to living healthy is to lead a healthy lifestyle. The body has its own mechanism to regenerate its machinery and regulate its circadian rhythm. Intake of frequent meals with refined sugar encourages glucose storage that subsequently leads to an insulin spike. Insulin spike is detrimental to the body and causes damage to blood vessels, vital organs and nerves. Poor eating habit also interferes with the digestion process and causes sleep abnormality. Sleep abnormality inhibits the release and action of the growth hormone, which is vital for the maintenance and regeneration of the organs of our body. Therefore, following a 10-hour eating window can improve glucose and lipid metabolism thereby enhancing

GH's activity, which can subsequently maintain the regeneration and functioning of the body system. In addition to the same, involving in some form of physical activity such as brisk walking or engaging in a sport, of a personal choice, can help us remain healthy and disease-free.

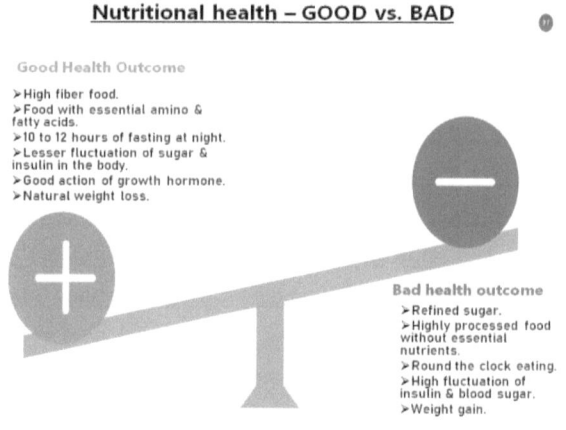

Figure 03: Showing nutritional habits; good health outcome vs. bad health outcome.

Quick Tip:

Therefore, for a healthy life, one should:

✓ Base every day meals on <u>high fibre carbohydrates</u> (both insoluble and soluble), <u>essential fatty acids</u> (Omega-3 fatty acid and Omega-6 fatty acid), and <u>essential amino acids</u> (Histidine, Isoleucine, Leucine, Lysine, Methionine, Phenylalanine, Threonine, Tryptophan and Valine). We should also eliminate refined and processed carbohydrate from the everyday diet. The essential fatty acids and amino acids are required because the human body is not equipped to produce it naturally. The high-fibre carbohydrates cannot be broken down into sugar molecules, and instead help to regulate blood glucose, check hunger, and facilitate improved digestion.

- ✓ Consume abundant fruits and vegetables as they are a rich source of vitamins and minerals.
- ✓ Eliminate sugary food and saturated fat, and
- ✓ Consume unsaturated fat.
- ✓ Restrict consumption of salt to only 6g per day, for adults.
- ✓ Consume oily fishes that are a source of omega-3 fatty acids.
- ✓ Never skip breakfast.
- ✓ Consume 6 to 8 glasses of water every day.
- ✓ Lead a physically active lifestyle and devote time to brisk walking and regular exercising.
- ✓ A short discussion on Tea, Coffee, and Chocolates:

Benefits:

The most common beverages consumed, after water, include tea and coffee. The popular drinks contain caffeine that acts as a stimulant to the central nervous system. Caffeine has been studied to reduce fatigue, drowsiness, improve concentration and improve motor coordination. In addition to the same, coffee beans and tea leaves also contain antioxidants that lower the risk of cardiovascular diseases and cancer. Intake of antioxidants also prevents the damage caused to the body due to oxidation. Dark chocolates made up of 60% cacao contain approximately 20 mg of caffeine in every 1.5 ounces of serving. Dark chocolates are also a rich source of caffeine and comprise all the health benefits stated above.

- The Problem and the Solution:

The caffeine present in the tea, coffee, or dark chocolate has a life of 5 to 6 hours. It means that only after the passing of 5 to 6 hours can the body effectively eliminate one-half of the caffeine consumed. So, ideally, the consumption of caffeinated substances is recommended 8 hours before bedtime. That would ensure that the sleep remains undisturbed. Undisturbed sleep, in turn, enables the regeneration and restoration activity of the GH to remain undisturbed. Also, caffeinated beverages must not be consumed with sugar, but can be consumed with substitutes such as honey/ jaggery, as the addition of sugar eliminates the beneficial properties of caffeine.

✓ **A short discussion on alcohol:**

- Alcohol, when consumed in a moderate dose, has proven to have health benefits. The average amount recommended is one drink for women and up to two drinks for men. The following examples better define the meaning of one drink:

    Beer: 12 fluid ounces (355 ml)

    Wine: 5 fluid ounces (148 ml)

    Distilled Spirits (80 proof): 1.5 fluid ounces (44ml)

    Consumption of alcohol in the recommended doses has been proven to reduce risks of cardiovascular diseases, reduce risks of ischemic stroke and the risk of developing diabetes.

- The problem and solution:

Alcohol has a shorter life of 2 hours. This means the body requires 2 hours to metabolize the consumed alcohol. Therefore, drinking alcohol right before bedtime interferes with a peaceful sleep that inhibits GH's action. Consumption of alcohol is recommended 2 hours before sleep. Spirits of any type must be consumed along with 250 ml of water. Drinking water with alcohol slows down the absorption rate, facilitating improved metabolism of the alcohol in the body.

✓ **A short discussion on Smoking:**

Smoking, however, is not good at all. It stimulates the brain to release a chemical substance called "dopamine." It promotes the "feel-good" factor to people, especially those suffering from anxiety and/ or depression. The "feel-good" factor is the initiation of the vicious circle of nicotine addiction. Lack of nicotine curtails the "feel-good" factor that causes withdrawal syndromes such as irritability, anxiety and craving. That consequently transforms into an addiction. Smoking has no proven health benefits. It has been confirmed to cause different kinds of cancer, lung and respiratory diseases and increases the risks of acquiring multiple chronic disorders such as stroke, heart attack, diabetes, and hypertension.

✓ **Morning rituals to kick start the day with –**

- Drink at least one litre of water in the morning.
- Drinking stomach lemon juice or apple cider vinegar, on an empty stomach, is very healthy.

- Sun exposure for at least fifteen minutes.
- Full body exercise for 15 to 20 minutes, before you take your breakfast.
- Meditate for at least 5 minutes. Sit in a relaxed posture, close your eyes, and just become mindful about your breath. Concentrate between your eyebrows (the seat of your CEO – the most advanced part of your brain – the prefrontal cortex).
- Practice being grateful for the past, present and the future.
- Practice expanding the light of bliss and love to the universe.
- Become mindful of the critical things you want to achieve.
- Always visualize positive and beautiful things.
- Have your bath regularly, and be in the present while doing so. Enjoy bathing and bring varieties in your soap, shower gel, etc. Sing and enjoy the bathing process.
- Then eat a high protein & high fibre breakfast. Munch on some nuts like walnuts, almonds and peanuts.
- A full cup of black coffee is welcome.
- Focused and mindfulness in socialization with your family is a perfect option at the breakfast table.

- If you still have some time left, you can write a journal about the essential things or focus on the critical issues that require your focused attention.

Let our body settle down with the natural food and eating window. Supply your body with essential nutrients, and it will readjust it's metabolism to natural and unprocessed food. It will take around eight to ten weeks to adjust the metabolism to the proper eating window and the intake of whole natural foods. With some exercise, for 15 to 30 minutes a day by your side, and adequate sleep, you will own excellent health and a resilient body. Now weight loss and gain will not be a problem. Keeping your body in its natural weight and shape is far more comfortable than the natural food and eating window. The change that you will make will start showing after three months of achieving healthy living. Let's achieve excellent health by creating a new lifestyle around our healthy habits. It is doable and sustainable. I will discuss about sleep and exercise in the forthcoming chapters.

Keep this knowledge by your side when you eat food. Please, do not bring unsustainable solutions like "diet" or "supplements" or "extreme exercise at the gym" to your health. Follow a healthy lifestyle which is feasible to you and own it as your own for the sake of your life. Your body is what you eat and when you eat (the time window). Bring variety and creativity in your food with whole natural foods, which are full of essential nutrients. Be creative and enjoy this newly acquired lifestyle. Then, you can also become the guide and role-model for others, as a bright example of healthy eating and healthy living. You can be creative with healthy food ingredients that are mentioned in these chapters. Bring variety to the food that you consume. And I wish you the best of luck for that.

Table 01 Organic Sources of Essential Nutrients		
Name of the essential nutrients	**Few Benefits**	**Few Food items**
1. Essential Fatty Acids	- Essential component of our cell membrane - Improves our heart health - Reduces depression - Reduces inflammation - Decreases fatty liver - Promotes bone health - Promotes brain development - Building block of many essential body chemicals	• Sunflower seeds • Walnut • Almond • Cashew nut • Chia seeds • Flax seeds • Olive oil • Fish oils
2. Essential Amino Acids	- Enzyme formation	• Whole wheat • Whole rice • Whole maize

		- Important building blocks for almost all of the body's chemicals - Forms our muscle - Promotes mental alertness - Reduces depression	• Legumes • Egg • Chicken • Milk
3.	The fibre rich carbohydrates	- Improves insulin resistance - Improves digestion - Reduces constipation - Good for our immunity - Bring the goodness of essentials with it	• Cauliflower • Broccoli • Kidney beans • Chickpeas • Beetroot, • Mushrooms • Bell pepper • Celery • Cabbage • All green vegetables • Egg plant • Wheat bran • Sweet potatoes • Oats • Banana • Grapefruit • Apples • Oranges • Blue berries

Table No. 02 Organic Sources of Vitamins

Name of the VITAMINS	Few Benefits	Few food items
Vitamin B Complex	- Essential component of almost all body chemicals - Necessary for producing proper health from immunity to skin health, from mental health to formation of our blood - It is necessary for our cellular division and formation of our genetic materials	• Whole grains (brown rice, barley, millet) • Meat (red meat, poultry, fish) • Eggs and dairy products (milk, cheese) • Legumes (beans, lentils) • Seeds and nuts (sunflower seeds, almonds) • Dark, leafy vegetables (broccoli, spinach, kai lan) • Fruits (citrus fruits, avocados, bananas)
Vitamin C	- Maintains overall health and functionality of our body - Essential for healing of our	• Guavas • Pineapples • Mangoes • Strawberries • Bell peppers • Kiwi

	body, and cartilage and blood vessel formation - Antioxidant	• Strawberries • Oranges • Papayas • Broccoli • Tomatoes • Kale, etc.
Vitamin A	- Formation and maintenance of soft tissue, skin, skeletal muscle and mucous membrane - Essential for vision	• Goat cheese • Butter • Cheddar • Carrots • Sweet potatoes • Spinach • Lettuce • Broccoli • Bell pepper • Hardboiled egg • Lamb liver • Beef liver • Cod-liver oil
Vitamin D	- Important for immunity - Important for calcium absorption, skin health & bone health.	• Spinach • Egg yolks • Cheese • Mushrooms • Orange juice • Oatmeal • Soybeans • White beans • Kale • Okra • Collards • Some fishes, like sardines, salmon, perch

		and rainbow trout
• Fatty fishes, like tuna, mackerel and salmon
• Foods fortified with vitamin D, like some dairy products, orange juice, soy milk, and cereals
• Beef liver, etc.
•
Vitamin E	- Antioxidant
- Build strong immune system
- Essential for cells to communicate with each other	• Sunflower seeds
• Almonds
• Peanuts
• Avocadoes
• Spinach
• Kiwi
• Broccoli
• Walnut
• Olive oil
• Shrimp
• Trout
• Goose meat
• Lobster
• Canola oil, etc.
Vitamin K	- Clotting vitamin – without it our blood would not clot.	• Kale
• Spinach
• Avocado
• Green peas
• Kiwi

| | | - Broccoli
- Cabbage
- Brussels sprout
- Beef liver
- Chicken,
- etc. |

Table 03 Organic Sources of Minerals

Name of Minerals	Function	Source examples
Iron	- Required for red blood cell formation - For immunity	- Beans and lentils
- Tofu
- Baked potatoes
- Pumpkin seeds
- Soybeans
- Cashews
- Dark green leafy vegetables such as spinach
- Fortified breakfast cereals
- Whole-grain and enriched bread

		- Chick peas
- Egg
- Red meat
- Liver, etc.
Calcium	- Helping to build strong bones and teeth
- Regulating muscle contractions, including your heartbeat
- Making sure blood clots normally	- Milk, cheese and other dairy foods
- Green leafy vegetables – such as broccoli, cabbage and okra, but not spinach
- Soybeans
- Tofu
- Soya drinks with added calcium
- Nuts
- Bread and anything made with fortified flour
- Fish where you can eat the bones – such as sardines and pilchards
Others micronutrients	- Essential for body's	- Bananas
- Cantaloupe
- Raisins

		chemical formation - Proper cellular functioning	• Nuts • Fish • Spinach and other dark greens • Black beans, • Peas • Almonds • All other sources that were mentioned earlier come packed with these micro-nutrients and micro minerals.

References:

Ahirwar, R. and Mondal, PR, 2019. 'Prevalence of obesity in India: A Systematic Review.' *Diabetes & Metabolic Syndrome: Clinical Research & Reviews,13*(1), pp.318-321.

Barnes, AS, 2012. 'Obesity and Sedentary Lifestyles: Risk for Cardiovascular Disease in Women.' *Texas Heart Institute Journal, 39*(2), p.224.

Bhutani, S., Klempel, M.C., Kroeger, C.M., Aggour, E., Calvo, Y., Trepanowski, J.F., Hoddy, K.K. and Varady, K.A., 2013. 'Effect of Exercising while Fasting on Eating Behaviours and Food Intake.' *Journal of the International Society of Sports Nutrition, 10*(1), p.50.

Courtemanche, C., Tchernis, R., and Ukert, B., 2018. 'The Effect of Smoking on Obesity: Evidence from a Randomized Trial.' *Journal of Health Economics*, 57, pp.31-44.

Healthline (2019).*20 Foods That Are Bad for Your Health*. [online] Healthline. Available at: https://www.healthline.com/nutrition/20-foods-to-avoid-like-the-plague#section1 [Accessed 31 Jan. 2020].

Healthline (2020).*9 Popular Weight Loss Diets Reviewed*. [online] Healthline. Available at: https://www.healthline.com/nutrition/9-weight-loss-diets-reviewed#section3 [Accessed 31 Jan. 2020].

IDF SEA (2019).*Members*. [online] Idf.org. Available at: https://idf.org/our-network/regions-members/south-east-asia/members/94-india.html [Accessed 31 Jan. 2020].

Jamshed, H., Beyl, R.A., Della Manna, D.L., Yang, E.S., Ravussin, E. and Peterson, C.M., 2019. 'Early Time-Restricted Feeding Improves 24-Hour Glucose Levels and Affects Markers of the Circadian Clock, Aging, and Autophagy in Humans.' *Nutrients*, *11*(6), p.1234.

Moro, T., Tinsley, G., Bianco, A., Marcolin, G., Pacelli, Q.F., Battaglia, G., Palma, A., Gentil, P., Neri, M. and Paoli, A., 2016. 'Effects of Eight Weeks of Time-restricted Feeding (16/8) on Basal Metabolism, Maximal Strength, Body Composition, Inflammation, and Cardiovascular Risk Factors in Resistance-trained Males.' *Journal of translational medicine*,*14*(1), p.290.

NHS.UK (2018).*8 tips for healthy eating*. [online] nhs.uk. Available at: https://www.nhs.uk/live-well/eat-well/eight-tips-for-healthy-eating/ [Accessed 31 Jan. 2020].

Prabhakaran, D., Jeemon, P. and Roy, A., 2016. 'Cardiovascular Diseases in India: Current Epidemiology and Future Directions.' *Circulation*, *133*(16), pp.1605-1620.

Verywell Mind (2019).*How Alcohol Impacts Your Nutrition*. [online] Verywell Mind. Available at: https://www.verywellmind.com/nutritional-effects-of-alcohol-63192 [Accessed 31 Jan. 2020].

Weltman, A., Weltman, J.Y., Watson Winfield, D.D., Frick, K., Patrie, J., Kok, P., Keenan, D.M., Gaesser, G.A. and Veldhuis, J.D., 2008. 'Effects of Continuous Versus Intermittent Exercise, Obesity, and Gender on Growth Hormone Secretion.' *The Journal of Clinical Endocrinology & Metabolism*,*93*(12), pp.4711-4720.

Zhang, H., Tong, T.K., Qiu, W., Zhang, X., Zhou, S., Liu, Y. and He, Y., 2017. 'Comparable Effects of High-intensity Interval Training and Prolonged Continuous Exercise Training on Abdominal Visceral Fat Reduction in Obese Young Women.' *Journal of Diabetes Research,2017*.

Exercise - The minimum maintenance work for our body

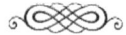

"Exercise is a celebration of what your body can do. Not a punishment for what you ate"

Anonymous

The term "exercise" triggers the image of a gym loaded with heavy equipment and people sweating on the treadmill and lifting heavyweight to get into the perfect body shape . . . does it not??

"Exercise," "fitness training," and "physical activity" seem hefty words that almost appear impossible for an average person to accomplish. The moment someone talks about fitness, the brain automatically starts thinking about a gym. However, the gym is not the answer to acquiring physical fitness. It's an industry, and it's not essential for a sustainable general fitness routine that a common man requires to be healthy.

Exercising and maintaining a healthy lifestyle can help to lead a life free from diseases and ailments. Exercising involves movement and utilization of all the body muscles, which in turn helps to maintain their functioning and keeps them in the best condition. Remember "all the muscles," must be a part of the process of exercise; both lower and upper body parts and both back and front. Also, the bigger the muscle is the higher the requirement of repetition. Our buttock and thigh muscles are more significant than our chest and arm muscles. Our back muscles are bigger than our abdominal muscles. So if you do sit-ups thirty times, you can exercise for biceps and triceps ten times. If you exercise your chest muscles ten times, do exercise which involves your back muscles thirty times. You can always start with five repetitions and then you can always scale up, weekly, by two more. At one go, you need to do more than ten repetitions. If you want to add some weight to your training - you can start adding dumbbells ranging from 1 kg up to 10 kg into your workout. You can do separate sets of muscles-workout every alternate day. But exercise with some weight training to all your muscles at least three times a week. That's the essential maintenance work that our body needs. And these activities can be done quickly at home with two dumbbells.

The ordinary benefits of aerobic exercises are as follows:

- An increased parasympathetic tone, which improves our circulation and reduces the chances of heart and its related diseases.

- Increased growth hormone level – more regeneration, more immunity and less stress on the body. There is lesser insulin resistance and lower chances of blood sugar and cholesterol related problems.

- Increase in GH (growth hormone) promotes a good appetite and digestive system.

- Increased muscle tone helps us to maintain proper posture and thus reduces muscle pains here and there. Joints and bones also remain healthy with higher bone-mineral density and lower incidence of osteoporosis.

- Exercise increases the levels of dopamine, endorphins, anandamide, etc. in the brain. These elevate mood and helps in motivation, thus increasing focus.

- It kick-starts our circadian rhythm in the morning and, with some exercise in the afternoon, it boosts our evening performance. Thus promoting excellent sleep.

There are many other benefits as well, which has not been mentioned here.

However, despite the benefits of exercise, when a physician recommends exercise for leading a healthy life, the most common responses are:

"Umm . . . I don't have the time to hit the gym' or "The gym next-door is costly. I cannot afford the registration fees" or "I am a senior citizen and am too old for the gym" or "Exercise does not make sense, I would prefer to go on a diet instead" or "I am already slim, why do I need to exercise?"

You will be able to dismiss the myths associated with exercise and fitness by the end of the chapter. You will, also, be able to understand the true essence of fitness.

The beliefs that need to be changed:

"Healthy is an outfit that looks good on everybody" - Anonymous.

"Physical fitness" is equivalent to being healthy, and it does not require the gym. Strict dieting, taking of supplements, engaging in rigorous workout, or starving to be slim is not relevant to physical fitness. Those are industries and have some importance for athletes, but these are not required for the purpose of general fitness. Exercising is not just "heavy-weight lifting" or "100 push-ups" in the gym to get six-pack abs. These are simply advertisements clouding your judgment.

In the rawest sense, being healthy requires maintaining a healthy lifestyle and activating every muscle's function to ensure improved health outcomes. Several research studies have revealed the benefits of exercising regularly. Exercising not only helps with weight management but also accelerates the rate of metabolism. It improves cardiac output, reduces the risk of high blood pressure and strengthens the functioning of the immune system. Further, it has also been studied to increase self-esteem, boost energy levels and strengthen bones and joints. Exercise and physical fitness have further been considered to improve self-image, promote the toning of muscles, and alleviate stress. With so many evidenced benefits of exercise and physical fitness, does it still seem impractical and irrelevant to exercise regularly?

"Exercise is healthy for you!" We have all heard this phrase a million times. Somehow, our will to exercise and lead a healthy lifestyle is overshadowed by the problems of unfortunate exercising habits, consumption of an unhealthy diet and the leading of a sedentary lifestyle. Time and again, several research studies have proven the advantages that are associated with regular exercise. Exercise helps to manage body weight and prevents obesity; to manage and control body weight, we need to burn the calories that are consumed by us. When an individual cannot burn the number of calories consumed, the calorie gets stored in the body and adds to the body fat. Exercise improves motor neuron activity and prevents risks of falls in the elderly. It improves mental health and mood, reduces the chances of colon cancer, breast cancer, uterine cancer, or lung cancer, and effectively regulates the blood sugar level. Exercise improves people's quality of sleep and efficiently maintains their biological clock or circadian rhythm (the daily hormonal and functional ups and downs inside our body).

Exercising helps to lower the blood sugar level and ensures better functioning of the insulin hormone. This helps to reduce the risk of acquiring metabolic Type II Disease. Also, exercise helps to strengthen the circulatory system and the cardiac output, thereby increasing the blood's oxygen level and reducing the risk of problems such as coronary artery disease or hypertension.

Therefore, from the data collected and from the evidence received, it can be stated that exercise is hugely beneficial for the body. However, not every type of exercise is healthy for the body. Exercise only benefits the body when it is done correctly. Thus it is essential to understand the three training components, which include intensity, timing and type.

Exercise Intensity:

Research studies recommend that exercising regularly is equivalent to 60% of the total heart rate - age-specific heart rate = (220-Age) - for 20 min to an hour per day is beneficial for health. Research has recommended that regular exercise is equivalent to 60% of the total heart rate. The age specific heart rate can be calculated by subtracting your age from 220 (220-age). Exercising from 20 minutes to an hour is thus beneficial to your health. These are aerobic exercises. While exercising, if you can talk a simple sentence properly – you are doing aerobic activity.

Any intense exercise which lasts for more than an hour per day and where the heart rate is more than 70% will make the exercise anaerobic; it will bring the stress hormone "cortisol" into the play and reduce the functioning of growth hormone. Thus it is less beneficial for the body.

In the case of high-intensity workout (HIIT), when more or equal to 90% of the total heart rate can be achieved, it is recommended that exercising for 20 to 45 seconds for 2 to 3 times per week is beneficial for the body. But while doing regular aerobic exercises, all body muscles are required before aiming for HIIT. The body should be adequately hydrated and nourished with natural and whole foods. Recovery and sleep should be taken proper care of. Remember, when you do exercise, you break the muscles and when you sleep or rest the muscles, you build it. So sleep is very important.

Any exercise beyond the discussed intensity would harm the body as it would release the stress hormone, cortisol. This would subsequently inhibit the growth hormone and prevent active regeneration of the muscle and body functions.

Timing for Exercise:

The best time to exercise is in the morning after drinking 1 litre of water. Research studies mention that exercising or working out after 12 hours of fasting, increases the GH activity and improve insulin sensitivity, which in turn assists with enhanced body functions.

Afternoon exercise has also been suggested to be beneficial for the body. But exercising should be avoided either before the meal, after the meal, or 2 to 3 hours before bedtime. If you exercise just before bedtime, it results in the release of the brain's dopamine. This induces motivation but interferes with the ability to sleep peacefully at night.

Exercise Type:

It is recommended that about 20 to 30 minutes of aerobic exercise helps to achieve 60% of the total heart rate, which is beneficial for health. This can blend sit-ups and also involve all the muscles for a weight-training with dumbbells. Playing a sport such as cricket, football or badminton also includes movement of all muscles (that means all body muscles; do not forget the muscles of thighs, buttocks and back when you select your activity). HIIT or high-intensity workout is not recommended regularly and is only beneficial for health if done up to three times a week up to a maximum of 45 seconds.

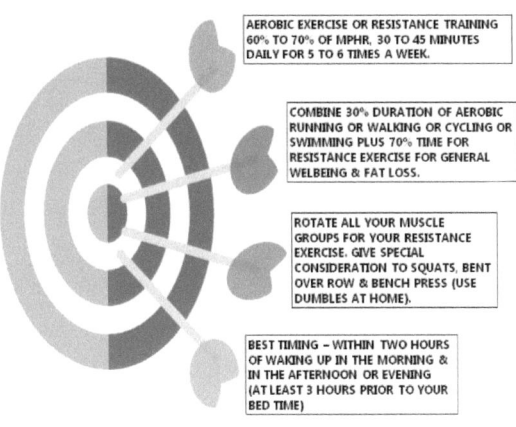

Figure 04: Showing the ideal timing, types and duration of exercise for optimal health benefits.

The solution:

The results of leading a sedentary lifestyle are frightening and documented within the evidence base to be chronic illnesses. People with a reduced level of physical exercise are at a high risk of fatal health problems such as diabetes, heart disease, Alzheimer's disease, premature death, etc. Sedentary lifestyle and inactivity can worsen the symptoms of arthritis and increase low back pain; it can also cause anxiety, moodiness, and loss of focus. The gift of life is beautiful and if doing a bit can help us relish it, then why should we not devote time to nurture the gift of life?

The science behind the solution:

The solution to health problems such as Type II diabetes, obesity, hypertension, cardiovascular disorder, PCOS, PCOD and arthritis is exercising regularly, consuming a healthy diet and living an active lifestyle. Exercising daily helps to improve the function of Growth Hormone, stimulate the impact of dopamine in the brain, increase insulin sensitivity, kick-start the circadian rhythm that facilitates a peaceful sleep at night and promote better regeneration of the body. In addition to the same, it also improves memory function, blood circulation, mental health outcomes and helps in improving digestion and absorption. Therefore, exercising should be mandatory for each one of us to stay healthy and lead longer lives.

Quick tips:

Some quick tips that can help each one of us stay happier and healthier:

4. Improve the hydration status of your body.
5. Provide your body the nourishment of natural whole grain and whole foods. Avoid fried and processed food, including refined sugar.
6. Include more Omega 3 fatty acids and essential amino acids in your diet.
7. Avoid taking food at night for at least 12 hours to own a healthy lifestyle.
8. Sleep and recover for at least for seven hours a day.
9. Then start exercising in the morning.

10. Start with the aerobic activities for ten minutes. Then gradually build up to ten more minutes of exercise per day.
11. Avoid HIIT in the beginning. Once you can comfortably partake in aerobic exercises, for at least thirty minutes and have been doing so for almost a month, only then attempt HIIT.
12. Avoid exercising just after meals, for at least two hours.
13. Avoid exercising 2 hours before bedtime as it hampers sleep.
14. Exercise in comfortable clothes.
15. Consume 500 ml of water as you start exercising and a litre of water slowly in sips during and after the exercise.
16. Monitor your progress and set personalized and healthy goals.
17. You can opt to take vitamin C and vitamin B complex as supplements when you start exercising.
18. Keep yourself motivated.

Move your sub-conscious and stop procrastinating –

The process: Now, the uninstalling of the unproductive thoughts and simultaneously installing a productive idea is required. The actions to be taken are as follows –

Recognition:

Recognize clearly that not exercising is not helping you anymore. Practice to write journals as it's a great way to produce new thoughts and beliefs. Write in your journal, "Not exercising daily is causing me many problems . . ." Write down five to ten problems that it will create soon. "Exercise is highly productive for my long-term future because . . . " Write down five to ten facts about it. Read this every day after you wake up in the morning and at night before going to bed.

Declaration:

Write down in the journal, "I am an athlete with great physical fitness." Please write it down ten times. Then, read it, or if possible, repeatedly write it ten times in the morning and ten times before going to bed, daily. Also, whenever you talk to yourself, declare, "I am an athlete." Declare this positive thought to yourself, consciously again and again. You need to do these repetitive acts for two to three months. After that, the idea becomes hardwired; the app gets installed in our mind. Then you will become the thought. You will start thinking, behaving, and acting according to your new belief, even unknowingly.

Practise meditation and mindfulness to overcome the procrastination towards exercise.

When you write in your journal, the science behind it is focused on and it produces muscle memory by creation of the thoughts and the experience of writing them simultaneously. When you repeat the process again and again, it accelerates the process of formation of a new neural net inside your brain for your new habit.

Keep doing it, and you will start noticing the change within 2 to 3 months.

When we repeatedly declare things to our mind while being alert and awake, like who we are, it creates a new neural net about "who we are?" and prunes down the neural net of "who we are not." The declarative memory with repeated experience gradually becomes hardwired in our brain.

When we visualize things vividly with strong emotions – we form a memory. We already discussed that we could recreate any event in our mind without it happening, and it creates the same response in the brain and our body as if it were occurring in real-time. When you wake up in the morning, your mental state is in alpha, and when you close your eyes, the brain quickly drifts into alpha brain waves. Remember, alpha is the bridge between our conscious and subconscious mind. So, learning happens faster when we are in alpha. When you begin visualizing and adding emotions to the visualization, like the feeling of pain, frustration, motivation, happiness, etc., you start producing the theta. You begin forming a new memory for yourself with the help of your temporal lobe and hippocampus. The repeated firing of these new neural bundles is hardwired in our brain and thus in our subconscious. This thought is then automated. Now the idea will start firing in spite of you. Therefore you install new habits. It may become challenging for you not to exercise regularly. However, as you are virtually no longer using the old unproductive neural net, it will prune away. Thus, the older unproductive belief is uninstalled.

I am not telling the journey will be smooth and easy, and that you will not fail in the way. I guarantee you that you will fail repeatedly. But it doesn't matter. The start will be jerky, then it will seem chaotic, but when you reach your goal, it will feel incredible. Just keep on doing things, and as you go ahead, the progress gradually becomes more effortless. The next change will be far more natural; the third change will be even easier. You will be able to develop the muscle of change within you. You can become the personality that you want to grow into; one which serves you better as and when required.

Be creative in your journey.

References:

Akins, J.D., Crawford, C.K., Burton, H.M., Wolfe, A.S., Vardarli, E. and Coyle, E.F., 2019. 'Inactivity Induces Resistance to the Metabolic Benefits Following Acute Exercise.' *Journal of Applied Physiology*, 126(4), pp.1088-1094.

Fiuza-Luces, C., Santos-Lozano, A., Joyner, M., Carrera-Bastos, P., Picazo, O., Zugaza, J.L., Izquierdo, M., Ruilope, L.M. and Lucia, A., 2018. 'Exercise Benefits in Cardiovascular Disease: Beyond Attenuation of Traditional Risk Factors.' *Nature Reviews Cardiology*, 15(12), pp.731-743.

Mandolesi, L., Polverino, A., Montuori, S., Foti, F., Ferraioli, G., Sorrentino, P. and Sorrentino, G., 2018. 'Effects of Physical Exercise on Cognitive Functioning and Wellbeing: Biological and Psychological Benefits.' *Frontiers in Psychology*, 9, p.509.

Nystoriak, M.A. and Bhatnagar, A., 2018. 'Cardiovascular Effects and Benefits of Exercise.' *Frontiers in Cardiovascular Medicine*, 5, p.135.

Spiegelman, B. ed., 2017. *Hormones, Metabolism, and the Benefits of Exercise*. Springer.

Wasser, J.G., Vasilopoulos, T., Zdziarski, L.A. and Vincent, H.K., 2017. 'Exercise Benefits for Chronic Low Back Pain in Overweight and Obese Individuals.' *PM &R*, 9(2), pp.181-192.

Recovery and Sleep

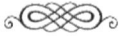

"Life is not merely being alive, but being well."

-Marcus Valerius Martialis

Sleep is vital and an integral part of our health. Research reports mention that insufficient sleep has emerged to be a common health issue that affects 25% of U.S. adults. Research data within the Indian context also states that approximately 93% of India's population are sleep deprived and can manage less than 8 hours of recommended sleep. Also, 58% of those affected by lack of sleep have reported poor performance at work and a diminished quality of life. Hence, based on the available research data, it can be said that the situation is complicated and must be looked into, immediately, to promote wellness outcomes for the general population.

Wrong beliefs about our sleep

The big problem here is our wrong beliefs about our sleep.

Sleep is the most compromised element in our daily life. We think that sleep can easily be sacrificed as and when required.

Most of us are under the impression that lack of sleep yields higher productivity. Some of us also consider rest as a waste of time.

We do not believe that the physical exercise that we do in the morning or the afternoon has nothing to do with our sleep quality. **

The importance of exposure to sunlight for at least an hour during daytime is also wholly forgotten. **

Our thoughts that are carried out daily determine our sleep quality at night (ideas that do not give rise to any productive action should be avoided at will).

The same is applicable for our food quality and our eating window. **

We hold the wrong idea that bedrooms can be used for many activities, and which does not affect our sleep. The bedroom should be a visual input for relaxation and sleep.

The bedroom ambiance (light, sound, and smell), the mattress and pillow also determine our sleep quality.

** These activities boost our circadian rhythm and thus produce excellent sleep quality.

Each of the existing wrong beliefs and misconceptions should be acknowledged. Then we have to become mindful of what activities we perform when are awake to promote good sleep quality. Thus our body and brain will recover better for high performance daily. A healthy lifestyle is a myth without the truth of sleep present in it. Every aspect of sleep is essential, ranging from an almost fixed bedtime to mattress and pillow quality. The bedroom ambiance, what we eat and drink throughout the day, the physical exercise that we do regularly and what we think every moment, all of this directly affects our sleep quality. In accordance to a report published by the *Medical News Today*, it has been stated that low sleep quality and acute deprivation of sleep is associated with several health concerns such as a weak immune system and has a direct impact on the overall body weight. It also negatively affects the level of blood pressure that can increase the risk of acquiring cardiovascular diseases and hormonal imbalance. In addition to the same, sleep deprivation also results in general symptoms such as fatigue, lack of concentration, reduced productivity, inducing forgetfulness and other issues related to a poor mental health outcome.

The little science of circadian rhythm

We have a clock embedded in our brain (in the hippocampus), which regulates the hormonal changes in our body; it maintains our daytime wakefulness and active state, and night-time sleep recovery. The sunlight at daytime secretes melatonin by stimulating our receptors inside our eyes and causing a state of alertness. The hippocampus has a direct connection with our eyes. Thus, it knows when it's a day and when it's night. When we wake up, hormones like adrenaline, corticosteroids and sex hormones are at its peak. The insulin hormone is also secreted in our pulse at around 8 am. As the day progresses, these hormone levels come down and maintain a relatively lower level. As night comes, the sunlight fades away, causing the melatonin level to go down. In turn, the adenosine (the sleep chemical which gets blocked by coffee) level, in the brain, increases. Other stimulatory hormones also come down. We feel tired and fall asleep. Sleep is necessary for the recovery and regeneration of our body. It also restores the brain chemicals for the proper functioning of our mind, for the next day. It is only at night, when we sleep, that the new neural synapses are formed, and neural networks are hardwired. So, the biological clock that maintains our sleep and wake cycle also helps us to function regularly with less stress.

A short story from our daily life:

Cecelia is a 27-year-old, confident and charming woman who has recently been an ABC firm operations manager. Her office schedule does not give her much time to do what she loves to do the most i.e. watch her favourite movies and web-series. With her everyday schedule being tightly-packed, she decided to catch up on her favourite shows post-dinner until the wee hours of the morning. Camelia, her flatmate, would often tell her to get a good night's sleep to be healthy, but Cecelia would choose to ignore it. Every day after dinner, Camelia asked Cecelia not to watch movies until late at night. She cited her elder sister's example, whose health had started deteriorating due to a lack of sleep. However, Cecelia would get angry and ask Camelia not to lecture her about her health. Camelia gradually stopped sharing her concern because of Cecelia's reaction.

Meanwhile, Cecelia would have a decadent dinner and sip on an espresso while watching her favourite shows until 4 am on a bright screen. She would then struggle to sleep, and when 8 am came, she would struggle to get up and report to her office. Cecelia has been following this routine for more than six months now and has lost weight. She looks unwell and underweight and has fainted twice at her office because of low blood pressure. She can feel her productivity is drastically going down and this has been highlighted by her immediate reporting manager.

Camelia, on the other hand, had been living a healthy lifestyle all the while. She would get up at 7 am; go for a jog for 20 minutes, before freshening up and reporting to her office by 9 am. She works in a different firm as an accountant and would generally be back home by 6 pm. She would then have her dinner by 9 pm following which she would usually fall asleep by 10 pm. She would wake up in the morning energized and feel her best. Over the previous six months, she has delivered her best performance and is also healthy.

Cecelia decided to see her general physician for her poor health. Her general physician assessed her condition and told her that she is sleep-deprived. Cecelia now reflects on what Camelia often told her and compares her present situation with Camelia's current state. She realizes the importance of sleep and of leading a healthy lifestyle. She loses her calm and bursts into tears and starts anticipating if it is too late. . .

The science behind the story:

Our body requires seven hours of sleep in order to complete the sleep-wake cycle Two hours of sound sleep are needed in three repetitions with half an hour for entering into the sound sleep phase and half an hour to come out of the sound sleep phase. During the night, the level of melatonin (a hormone) in the body increases thereby promoting sleepiness. The hormone melatonin is found naturally within the body. It plays a vital role in regulating the sleep-wake cycle and the biological clock or the body's circadian rhythm. The production of this hormone is directly dependent on the absence of light and therefore, for the same reason, the hormone level, within the body, is high at night. During the day, the level of melatonin production in the body decreases sharply and as a result, the body is prepared to be alert and active. The fact that Cecelia binge watches her favourite shows on her laptop, using a bright light filter, is responsible for enhancing the level of melatonin hormone, which inhibits her sound sleep at night.

As it has already been discussed in the previous chapter, the consumption of caffeinated beverages promotes alertness. Caffeine is a stimulant that acts as an 'adenosine receptor agonist' and thus inhibits sleep. Adenosine is a naturally occurring chemical within the body that plays a vital role in energy production and affects sleep. Adenosine promotes sleepiness. Consumption of caffeine results in the blocking of the adenosine receptors within the body, thus keeping the body from falling asleep. Hence, Cecilia's excessive use of coffee can be explained as another reason that interfered with her ability to enter into sound asleep.

Also, the consumption of a heavy meal at night interferes with the ability to sleep peacefully. Eating a heavy meal before bedtime causes an insulin spike and also increases the risk of suffering from indigestion or GERD (Gastroesophageal reflux disease); this inhibits a sound sleep. REM (rapid eye movement) sleep is necessary for the body to regenerate itself, and a peaceful sleep promotes the action of the Growth Hormone to repair and restore the body. There have been studies which mention that gut flora also regenerates and replenishes itself, only when the body sleeps soundly. Hence, late-night snacking and the consumption of a heavy meal can be attributed to Cecelia's low sleep quality that has now taken a toll on her health.

Poor quality sleep is associated with the triggering of obesity, diabetes, hypertension, anxiety, weak immunity and several other physical and mental health disorders. Poor sleep or lack of sleep disturbs the natural biological clock or the circadian rhythm of the body. This, in turn, results in reduced productivity and poor efficiency. Therefore a sound sleep is essential to lead a healthy life.

The solution:

> "Health is the first muse,
>
> and sleep is the condition
>
> to produce it."
>
> *- Ralph Waldo Emerson*

Cecelia needs to adapt to a healthy lifestyle and good bedtime habits in order to lead a life which would remain free from illnesses. First and foremost, she must stop overtly stressing herself in her workplace. Followed by that, she must cut down on her consumption of coffee; she must ensure that her last cup of coffee is at least 6 to 8 hours before bedtime, so as to not disturb her sleep. She must also avoid binge-watching her shows until the wee hours of the morning and adapt a bedtime routine. She must prevent consuming a heavy dinner, and if there is a need to work on her laptop or use her cell phone at night, she must start using the "blue-light filter." She must engage in mild exercise such as brisk walking for 15 to 20 minutes to help her sleep peacefully. It is advised that engaging in mild exercise is equivalent to the utilization of the 60% of the maximum permissible heart rate (220 minus Age is the formula) and that can ensure sound sleep at night.

The science behind the solution:

Coffee contains caffeine that blocks the adenosine receptors, which promotes the feeling of sleepiness. It is because of this reason that consumption of any form of caffeine, such as tea, coffee and dark chocolate must be avoided for at least 8 hours before bedtime. Caffeine has a half-life of approximately 3 to 5 hours in the body. It means that caffeine's impact remains within the body for a more extended period after its consumption and interferes with the natural sleep-wake cycle.

On top of that, the intake of a substantial dinner results in an insulin spike. This spike in insulin increases the risk of GERD or gastrointestinal irritation. It inhibits the growth hormone's activity to restore and regenerate the body. The GH fails to function when the blood's insulin level is high; the body is acutely deprived of its repair mechanism.

Using a bright light filter has been studied to contribute to sleep problems. Electronic devices, such as laptops and cell phones, emit light ranging in the blue wavelength that tricks the brain into thinking that it is daytime. The "blue light" interferes with the body's natural biological clock and causes downregulation adenosine production and activity, which consequently inhibits sleep.

Also, engaging in mild exercise has been studied to improve and increase sleep quality. Studies show, better sleep eliminates stress and anxiety. Gentle exercise, such as jogging in the morning, has been observed to boost deep sleep. Vigorous exercise should be avoided as it has been studied to be linked with insomnia. Spending time engaged in physical activity has been studied to increase the time duration for deep sleep, also known as the restorative sleep phase. The action of the GH is the highest while repairing and restoring the body of its wear and tear.

PROMOTE SLEEP- LAST 2 HOURS OF SLOW-DOWN

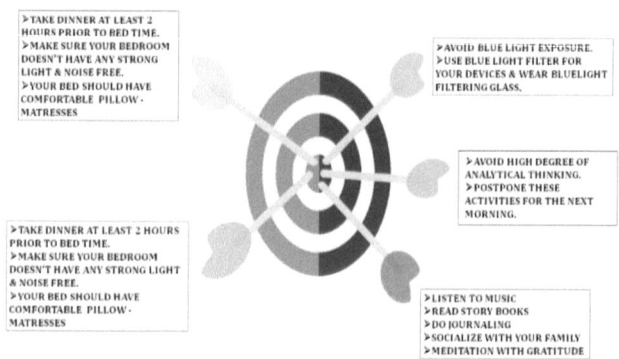

Figure 05: Showing the factors that promotes sleep in the last 2 hours before bed-time.

Quick tips:

Therefore for healthy sleep, one should:

- Kick-start your biological clock in the morning with 15 to 20 minutes of exercise, drinking one litre of water and exposure to sunlight for the same duration.

- You can also consider having sex in the morning hours as our sex hormones are at their peak during that time.

- A colder water bath is a welcome to start the day.

- If possible, a second dose of exercise and sunlight can also be taken in the afternoon.

- During the daytime, exposure to sunlight and physical activities for 15 to 45 minutes improves sleep at night.

- Avoid consuming caffeinated beverages and nicotine close to bedtime (6 to 8 hours of abstinence).

- A day-time short nap can be taken for half an hour max. Anything more than that is not suitable and will hamper sleep at night. A longer sleep can only be considered when you are compensating the sleep debt when you were awake the night before.

- Avoid heavy meals near bedtime (take dinner at least 2 hours before bedtime).

- Avoid using digital devices near bedtime for at least 2 hours – if you have to use them, please use them with blue light filter.

- Avoid exposure to bright light before bedtime, for at least 2 hours; you can use different lighting near bedtime or can also wear glasses with a blue light filter. Also, avoid blue light when you wake up in the middle of the night for any reason.

- Avoid brainstorming, high analytical and decision-making activities (if not an emergency) for at least 2 hours before bedtime.

- A warm water bath or sauna is welcome at the day's end.

- Maintain a fixed bedtime routine plus or minus an hour.

- Ensure a pleasant sleeping environment in terms of ambiance like "no bright or blue lights," "no sound" and presence of "good smell" (essential oils are good).

- Use your bedroom mainly for sleeping and sexual activities.

- The quality of the mattress and pillow should also be on your mind, and you should consider changing them once in two to three years. (Remember you spend your life's one-third of the time sleeping.)

- Keep your food intake healthy with proper eating windows (already discussed).

- Keep your mind healthy with good productive living (already discussed).

- Meditation and mindfulness should be practised; to start and end the day with it is critical. Always add "gratitude" in your mindfulness and visualization program.

- Remember, the total sleep duration should be of seven hours. If any sleep debt is happening daily, try to compensate these with an afternoon nap and sleep heavily and for a longer time the next day.

More discussion on physical exercise can be found in the next chapter.

Take care of your sleep –

Your body and brain will regenerate and rejuvenate every night to ensure your high performance daily. Please use the ideas that we have discussed many times, earlier in the book, to move your sub-conscious. It will help you to overcome your belief barriers and proceed towards a healthier life. If you face problems and procrastinate while carrying out daily activities that yield a great sleep and recovery, use the following to move your sub-conscious:

Journaling

Write five long term health and performance issues that you will face if you do not follow quality sleep habits. Also, write down five good long term health and performance outcomes with good quality sleep.

Do mindfulness with visualization. Be mindful of the activities that you carry out throughout your day. Identify and avoid activities that are inhibiting your proper recovery and sleep at night.

References:

Colrain, I.M., Nicholas, C.L., and Baker, F.C., 2014. 'Alcohol and the Sleeping Brain.' *Handbook of Clinical Neurology* (Vol. 125, pp. 415-431). Elsevier.

Costello, R.B., Lentino, C.V., Boyd, C.C., O'Connell, M.L., Crawford, C.C., Sprengel, M.L. and Deuster, P.A., 2014. 'The Effectiveness of Melatonin for Promoting Healthy Sleep: A Rapid Evidence Assessment of the Literature.' *Nutrition Journal*, 13(1), p.106.

Gnocchi, D., and Bruscalupi, G., 2017. 'Circadian Rhythms and Hormonal Homeostasis: Pathophysiological Implications.' *Biology*, 6(1), p.10.

Goel, N., Basner, M., Rao, H., and Dinges, D.F., 2013. 'Circadian Rhythms, Sleep Deprivation, and Human

Performance.' *Progress in molecular biology and translational science* (Vol. 119, pp. 155-190). Academic Press.

Kervezee, L., Kosmadopoulos, A., and Boivin, D.B., 2018. 'Metabolic and Cardiovascular Consequences of Shift Work: The Role of Circadian Disruption and Sleep Disturbances.' *European Journal of Neuroscience.*

Mayo Clinic, 2020. Pros and cons of melatonin. [online] Mayo Clinic. Available at: https://www.mayoclinic.org/healthy-lifestyle/adult-health/expert-answers/melatonin-side-effects/faq-20057874 [Accessed 9 Feb. 2020].

Medic, G., Wille, M., and Hemels, M.E., 2017. 'Short and Long-Term Health Consequences of Sleep Disruption.' *Nature and Science of Sleep*, 9, p.151.

Medical News Today, 2020. 'Sleep deprivation: Causes, Symptoms, and Treatment. [online] Medical News Today. Available at: https://www.medicalnewstoday.com/articles/307334.php#effects [Accessed 9 Feb. 2020].

O'Callaghan, F., Muurlink, O., and Reid, N., 2018. 'Effects of Caffeine on Sleep Quality and Daytime Functioning.' *Risk Management and Healthcare Policy*, 11, p.263

Sleepfoundation.org 2020. 'What is Circadian Rhythm?' *National Sleep Foundation.* [online] Sleepfoundation.org. Available at: https://www.sleepfoundation.org/articles/what-circadian-rhythm [Accessed 9 Feb. 2020].

Stein, M.D., and Friedmann, P.D., 2006. 'Disturbed Sleep and its Relationship to Alcohol Use.' *Substance Abuse*, 26(1), pp.1-13.

Verywell Health, 2020. 'How Adenosine Helps You Get a Good Night's Sleep.' [online] Verywell Health. Available at: https://www.verywellhealth.com/adenosine-and-sleep-3015337 [Accessed 9 Feb. 2020]

Why stress management is important?

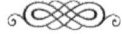

Stress is our coping response to the ever-changing world. In today's world the change is happening faster, but our evolution did not change much in last 100 years. So in the gap between our natural evolution and rapid changing environment, the lifestyle diseases are creeping in. We need to have strategies in place to use stress for bettering our performance. We have to prevent long-term stress and thus we need the coping strategies in place. That is why stress management is important.

How the emergence of temporary response "stress" can create cascades of long-standing problems in the human being?

That's the greatness about our brain.

When a rat sees a cat, it develops an immediate stress response and runs away from the place immediately. With the running away the stress response goes away, as well.

The rat cannot generate a stress response by visualizing the cat from its memory and projecting thoughts about the cat, when the cat is actually not there. It also cannot develop a neural circuit about a particular cat by repeatedly firing a bundle of neurons followed by the development of a self-sustained neural network. This network is one which can even fire spontaneously now and then with the mildest probability of the original stimulus at sub-conscious level, without even telling the rat.

We, humans, can do that. Thus, even in absence of the original stimulus we can continuously fire the neurons unknowingly and can produce the chemicals of stress. Now imagine that you have developed a 100 such neural nets due to a negative experience in the past and they fire every now and then with mildest predictive probability of the original event. But they do so without telling you. Thus, without your knowledge the stress button remains pressed for long time.

The following 10 changes happen in our body following long-standing stress:

1. Once our brain gets the stress signal, its hypothalamus (the controller of the hormonal system in our brain) starts producing hormone related to stress (CRH– Cortico-trophin releasing hormone). The stress releases the hormone from our pituitary gland (ACTH– Adreno-cortico Trophic Hormone) and this in turn releases adrenaline from our adrenal gland. In case of long term stress the hormone name glucocorticoid is increased.

2. The stress hormone prepares our body for a 3F response (Flight, Fight and Fright response).

3. It increases the body fuels that we would need for 3F- blood glucose level and the stored body fuel by means of cholesterol, etc.

4. It slows down our non-emergency but productive body activities i.e., digestion, regeneration and recovery.

5. It increases gastric acid secretions and causes palpitation, irritability, lack of sleep, depression, sexual dysfunction, headache, generalized body aches, etc.

6. It robs you of your dopamine system, your creativity and holistic thinking without the alpha activity in your brain; now you seek for addictions for the temporary escape from the situation, to the heavens of dopamine, at the cost of your health.

7. As in 3F mode our body puts away its vital energy source for excess body fuels by means of cholesterol.

8. It spends lesser energy on our immunity and regeneration process.

9. It increases chances of infections and degenerative diseases.

10. If it persists for a long time, it also can give rise to anxiety and panic disorders, diabetes, cholesterol problems, heart diseases, etc.

Why long-term stress is bad for our health

Stress is a natural mental and physical response to any demand. Any kind of challenge like productivity at work or school, an abrupt life change, or a psychologically painful event can be stressful. Stress can impact your health. It is vital to be sensitive about the handling of both minor and major causes of stress, so you're aware of when to look for assistance.

Here are some of the things you need to understand about stress:

1. Stress affects everyone.

Everyone experiences stress from time to time. Various types of stress exists, all of which contain a mental and physical health risk. Stress may be a short-term or a one-time incident, or it may repeatedly occur over a long period.

Examples of stress include:

- Regular stress is associated with pressure from family, work, school and other everyday duties.

- Stress resulting from an abrupt negative change such as sickness, break-up, death of a loved one, or losing a job.

- Traumatic stress resulting from events such as war, a dangerous accident, or natural calamity where individuals may be at the risk of suffering serious harm or even death. Individuals who suffer from traumatic stress may reveal deplorable temporary physical and emotional symptoms.

2. Not all stress is harmful.

In endangering situations, stress alerts the body to be ready to face a threat or run away for safety. In non-endangering situations, stress can motivate individuals, such as during examination or recruitment.

3. Long-term stress is bad for your health.

Dealing with the effects of chronic stress can be demanding. Given that long-term stress results from a regular stressor, compared to short-term stress, the body never gets a clear signal to regress to normal functioning.

Symptoms of chronic stress include:

- Headaches
- Irritability
- Insomnia
- Depression
- Anxiety

These are the most affected areas for individuals experiencing chronic stress:

• **Respiratory and cardiovascular systems**

In response to stress, you will experience rapid breathing to distribute oxygenated blood all through your body quickly. If you have pre-existing breathing problems such as emphysema or asthma, stress can make it even more difficult to breathe.

When stressed, your heart also pumps faster. Stress hormones lead to constriction of blood vessels directing more oxygen to your muscles, so that the muscles have enough strength to combat the situation. But this also raises your blood pressure, which increases the risk of heart attack and stroke.

• **Digestive system**

When stressed, your liver produces excess glucose to boost your energy. If you're experiencing chronic stress, your body may be unable to control this excess glucose rush. Chronic stress raises the risk of getting diabetes type 2.

Stress may also disrupt the way food moves through the body, causing constipation or diarrhoea. You might even have a stomach ache, vomiting, or nausea.

- **Reproductive system**

If stress persists for long, testosterone levels in a man begin to go down. This can tamper with sperm production resulting in impotence or erectile dysfunction. In females, stress can affect the menstrual cycle. It can result in more painful, heavier, or irregular periods.

- **Immune system**

Stress arouses the immune system which can be beneficial for immediate situations. This arousal can heal wounds and keep you away from infections. However, with time, stress hormones undermine your body's immune system making it ineffective. Individuals experiencing chronic stress are more prone to sicknesses like common cold and flu. Stress can also prolong the recovery time for an injury or an illness.

How an emergency quick response "stress" can create cascades of long-standing problems in the human being?

That's the greatness of our brain. When a rat sees a cat, it develops an immediate stress response and runs away immediately, following which the stress response goes out, too. The rat cannot generate a stress response by visualizing the cat from its memory. It cannot create thoughts about the cat when the cat is not there. The rat cannot develop a neural circuit about a particular cat by repeatedly firing a neuron bundle. It cannot build a prediction engine that can fire spontaneously now and then with the mildest probability of the original stimulus without its own knowledge (sub-conscious activity).

But you already know from the above discussions we can do that. Thus, even in the absence of the original stimulus, we can continuously fire the neurons unknowingly and produce stress. Imagine you have developed such 100 neural nets due to past negative experiences, and they fire every now & then with the mildest predictive probability of the actual event. And they do so without telling you. Thus, without your knowledge, the stress button remains pressed for a long time.

Now here are the cascades of events in our body – once our brain gets the stress signal. The hypothalamus (the controller of the hormonal system in our mind) starts producing hormones related to stress (CRH – Cortico-trophin releasing hormone). The CRH then releases the hormone from our pituitary (ACTH – Adreno-corticotropic Hormone), and this, in turn, releases adrenaline from our adrenal gland. The stress hormone prepares our body for a "3F" response (Flight, Fight & Fright response). It increases the body fuels that we would need for 3F mode - blood glucose level, stored body fuel through cholesterol, slows down our non-emergency but productive body activities, i.e., digestions, regeneration & recovery activities. It increases gastric acid secretions and causes palpitation, irritability, lack of sleep, depression, sexual dysfunction, headache, generalized body ache, etc. It robs you of your dopamine system. You are robbed of your creativity and holistic thinking without the alpha activity in your brain. Now you seek addictions for the temporary escape from the situation to the heavens of dopamine at your health cost. As in the "3F" mode, our body puts away its vital energy source for excess body fuels. It spends less energy on our immunity and regeneration process; thus, it increases infections and degenerative diseases. Persisting long, the "3F" or chronic stress mode can give rise to anxiety and panic disorders, diabetes, cholesterol problems, heart diseases, etc.

The Little Biology to Understand Stress

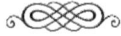

The term "stress" was coined by Hans Selye in 1936, who defined it as "the non-specific response of the body to any demand for change." Stress is the response generated by the body in the case of both negative and positive changes which occur in our environment. It is the coping mechanism to handle any new environmental change and life-threatening situation. But if chronically activated, it will alter our physiology negatively.

As a being of the highest evolution, we always seek reasons and purpose to do something. To uproot stress, we should learn our biology and understand the scientific explanations regarding the factors producing "stress," as dealt with in the later chapters. How should we handle them? What is the scientific basis for that? How is long-standing stress produced? How does long-term stress change our metabolism, chemical balance and immunity? Without knowing the reasons and purpose, we cannot go ahead with anything new. That's why the coming chapters will start the discussion with the gross relevant knowledge of our biology which will answer a lot of questions arising in our reasonable and purposeful mind. The biological knowledge that will be required to understand this book will be discussed that in three parts – Part I - The Psycho-neurology, Part II - Body in Chronic Stress.

Part I: Psycho-neurology –

The subconscious mind –

According to the famous psychologist Sigmund Freud, there are three levels at which the mind functions- the conscious, the preconscious, and the unconscious mind. The conscious mind is the one that defines all the actions as well as thoughts that occur when we are fully aware. The preconscious mind includes all the activities or reactions that happen automatically without giving too much thought. This includes driving a car, riding a bicycle, swimming, etc. However, we become aware of these actions as we think about them "consciously."

On the contrary, the unconscious mind is another layer of mind with all our memories and events. These things are usually inaccessible, no matter how much we try. These can be some of our childhood memories, such as the first time we tasted food or uttering a word and other similar things.

According to psychologists today, the subconscious mind can be a powerful tool to influence our behaviour. It is one of the most talked-about and researched subjects among psychologists around the world. The primary purpose of the subconscious mind is to make sure that we survive. It has a function called the homeostatic impulse, which regulates the body's essential functions, such as the body temperature, breathing and heartbeats. However, it is vital to note that apart from maintaining physical health, our subconscious mind also tries to regulate our mental health. Hence, it continually brings to our attention information and events that affirm our pre-existing beliefs. It again repeats similar thoughts to mimic things that we have already done in the past. In short, our subconscious mind keeps us in our comfort zones.

We, as a being, do 90% of our daily activity from the sub-conscious level. Can you remember how many times you brushed the teeth on your right-side today or what are obstacles you avoided when you walked through your house today? The answer to such questions will be "NO," almost always, if you are not consciously doing any new activity. At first, when you start a new activity, it requires the conscious effort to perform that activity. Then with repeated practice and feedback from experience, that skill (thought or action) becomes wired in your brain (new neural network is formed with a new memory in the brain. The cerebellum acquires that memory to put those in our automatic mind– the sub-conscious one). Now once it has been wired in our brain, it becomes automatic. Whenever required, our brain starts using that information even without telling us. If we go on doing the same thing again and again and live in the same place throughout our life, we will require a significantly less conscious effort (around 5%) to go through a typical day.

OUR MIND

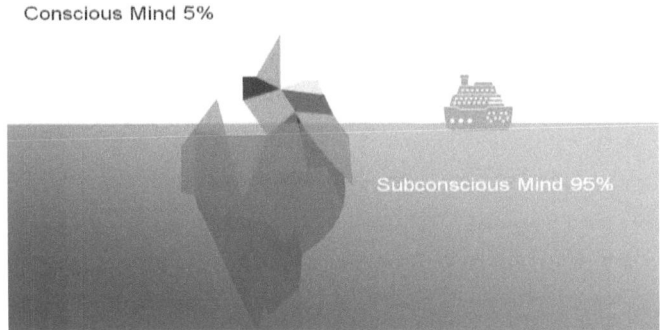

Figure 06: Showing 95% of our mind is automatic and is subconscious.

For example, remember that time when your house got renovated and the furniture was rearranged. You unknowingly got yourself injured for the first few times. However, with repeated practice, your subconscious acquires so much knowledge and experience about the environment that in a room packed with furniture and with significantly less lighting, you no more hurt yourself. The effort no more requires your conscious effort. By the same mechanism, singers can sing a song repeatedly, the swimmers can swim, the gymnast does the gymnastics, and the list is endless. We cannot analyse things or activities consciously and perform fluently and precisely but highly specialized activities. We cannot analyse things or activities consciously; however, to perform fluently and precisely we must rely on the conscious brain. Did you often notice you could not do something when you wanted to do it despite yourself? In such cases, we should firstly, distance ourselves from the subconscious so that our conscious and skilled activity to happen smoothly and effortlessly.

Like the same, you can repeatedly go back to a particular memory, say a negative and unproductive memory about a relative, say John. You often think that John always behaves rudely with you and never agrees with you even when you know nothing to disagree about. John never leaves any opportunity to cause you some embarrassment. Now you think consciously about why he is such a jerk around you a few times a day for 2 to 3 months. After that period, this memory, which is neither productive for you, nor it has any effect on John, gets hard-wired into your brain. With the slightest stimulation, like a person who looks a little like John or talks like John, you start feeling uncomfortable. When you go to a place where you are invited and there is a possibility of John being there as well, you start feeling that something is wrong. Even if a person is dressed like John, your brain starts firing those hard-wired neural networks even without telling you. You can mount the same amount of stress unknowingly at any point in time throughout your life, even without meeting John again.

1. Visualization and Emotional entanglement –

If you repeatedly visualize events, place, or person in your mind with robust emotional entanglement, you are hard-wiring your neural net. You create a neural net that will fire with the slightest probability of those things even without telling you. We should be cautious in what neural structure we build daily based on our memories and experiences. We should be aware that when these neural nets will be fired sub-consciously, it will not do any good to anyone on earth, irrespective of whether those will serve any good to ourselves or not.

2. The brain wave basic-

We know that our neurons send and receive messages by electrical activity in our body. And our brain has millions of neurons with around 150 trillion synapses. So, cumulatively, our brain produces electrical activities at various states of mind. We can also measure these activities by now employing EEG (electro-encephalogram). These waves are alpha, beta, gamma, theta, and delta.

The low-frequency beta wave represents sensory-motor activity at baseline for our muscles, other sensory activities and conscious alertness. The high-frequency beta wave represents stress and anxiety. The alpha is the bridge between beta, gamma on one side, and theta, delta on the other. Alpha is "the power of now." Without alpha, we are not using our subconscious store of wisdom and the computation power of our subconscious. Theta appears when we are in learning, memory formation, intuition, and in meditation and visualization mode. It is the doorway of the subconscious storehouse. Delta brainwaves occur during the deepest sleep without a dream and without self-awareness. It suspends external awareness ("ego") and is the source of empathy. Gamma wave represents the state of the brain when a different part of the brain is working simultaneously. The mind has to tone down high beta activity to access gamma. Gamma rhythm modulates perception and consciousness and it appears when we create new things and new thoughts.

Remember, without turning down the high beta activity of stress and anxiety you cannot access alpha and gamma. Thus, you cannot use "the power of now" and use your power of sub-conscious wisdom, creativity and calculations holistically. Remember, you work 90% from your sub-conscious mind daily. To train your sub-conscious, you need to access theta by repeated visualizations, thinking and activities. If you want to be creative, your beta activity should be minimized for your stress to be under control. Then you can have access to the gamma of creativity and lateral thinking. With a conscious, self-aware mind, we cannot access delta. For example, every evening, after work, you feel clumsy and exhausted with an increased reaction time and a component of irritability. The reason is the high beta activity and reduced alpha activity; gamma is not accessible at that time. But in the mornings your alpha activity is at its peak.

Chemical brain-

Our brain is also known as the "chemical brain," because it has many neuro-hormones that induce many states of mind and vice-versa. The highly exciting neurochemicals that we are going to discuss are - Dopamine, Serotonin, Nor-adrenaline, GABA (Gamma aminobutyric acid), Glutamate, Cannabinoids and Endorphins (endogenous morphine). Following are the chemicals and their gross functions in our brain –

a. **Dopamine-** This chemical is related to happiness, reward, and motivation. Every substance that creates addiction leads to the temporary release of dopamine and promotes substance abuse by spiralling up the need for the same response, as earlier. There are many states of mind and actions at which dopamine gets released in our brain without any external substance, i.e., new thoughts of curiosity, recent activities of interest, happiness in the now, exercise, positive visualization, etc. We feel motivated and pleased in this state of our brain. Did you feel motivated and happy traveling to new places, or learning new skills which you were curious about, or gaining some new knowledge? The answer, here, is probably "YES." Note that dopamine was secreted at these instances. You can also rob yourself of dopamine by sub-consciously running a negative and unproductive neural net about you and others (place, person and time). Remember, dopamine is the fuel and you are born motivated. Without it being activated sub-consciously, you may indulge in wrong dopamine release activities, i.e., overeating, becoming a shopaholic, irrationally being addicted to Facebook /

WhatsApp all night, or indulging in other e-commerce website searching for the sake of novelty. This wrongful release of dopamine, through harmful addictions, leads to dangerous consequences in terms of our health.

b. **Serotonin–** Causes massive effects on our mood. If you are sad and pessimistic about the world, your serotonin level decreases, and vice versa. And the result is bi-lateral; your elevated mood releases serotonin, and serotonin level will keep your mood elevated. More recent research confirms this. Hostility and negativity are associated not only with the development of heart disease but also with lower survival rates in the case of heart patients. The WHO's constitution states, "Health is a state of complete physical, mental and social well-being and not merely the absence of disease or infirmity." The positive mood, within the normal range, is a significant predictor of health and longevity. In a classic study, those in the lowest quartile for positive emotions, rated from autobiographies written at a mean age of 22 years, died on average ten years earlier than those in the highest quartile. We can release serotonin at will with self-induced positive mood, self-induced positive outlook about the world, an exposure to bright light, exercise, meditation and through food which is rich in tryptophan.

c. **Nor-adrenaline–** This neurotransmitter is one of the essential chemicals to be focused. It increases alertness, arousal, and decreases reaction time. The synthesis of nor-epinephrine depends on the presence of tyrosine, an amino acid found in proteins such as meat, nuts, and eggs. Dairy products such as cheese also contain high amounts of tyrosine (the amino acid is named "tyros," the Greek word for "cheese"). Tyrosine is the precursor to dopamine, which is in itself a precursor of epinephrine and nor-epinephrine. Banana peels contain significant amounts of nor-epinephrine and dopamine. So, when we increase the level of dopamine in the brain that in turn increases the nor-adrenaline level and therefore we can focus and be agile at work. The level of nor-epinephrine is reduced in our brain during depression. In an Alzheimer patient, 70% of nor-epinephrine receptors are lost. So, we should be doing activities to promote nor-epinephrine and dopamine to keep ourselves healthy.

d. **Glutamate**– It's an excitatory neurotransmitter that, on getting released, causes other neurons to fire. The neurochemicals are dopamine, serotonin, nor-adrenaline, etc.

e. **GABA (Gamma aminobutyric acid)**– It slows things down; it inhibits, and it dampens neural activity in the brain. The consumption of alcohol positively affects the GABA receptors in the brain to slow down brain activity and, at the same time, it increases dopamine. That brings pleasure without inhibitions but, of course, with harmful health consequences.

f. **Acetylcholine**– A neurotransmitter important for nerve conduction and plays an essential role in learning and memory formation.

g. **Cannabinoids**- Once these are activated, several pathways come into play. These result in a diverse array of effects, from the reduced experience of pain to the digestive tract movement and the impact on mood. In the hippocampus, they influence learning and memory. In the basal ganglia, they modulate locomotor activity and reward pathways. In the hypothalamus, they have a role in controlling appetite. Cannabinoids may also be protective against neurodegeneration and brain damage. It exhibits antiepileptic activity and analgesic effects.

h. Opioids- It is commonly used today to treat severe pain, for example, morphine (after Morpheus, the Greek god of dreams). The natural partners to the opioid receptors are the endorphins. These are released during certain activities, such as running (they are thought to be responsible for the 'runner's high'), regular exercise (75 to 150 minutes per week of moderate exercise), massage, chocolate consumption, chili- pepper consumption, sexual activity and pain. Other activities that release endorphins (endogenous morphine– morphine which is present in the body) are volunteering, donating, helping others, yoga and meditation.

If the brain chemicals seem a little overwhelming to you, remember the dopamine and serotonin for now. Remember, your brain's chemicals are not your goals to achieve; rather, they are the essential fuels to achieve your goals in life. Thus, the happiness, the motivation, the festive mood, the focus in the now, etc., that those chemicals induce are the biological needs for your brain to produce a healthy and productive mind. Also note that exercise, positive mood, proper food, helping others and meditation are the most common, scientifically proven, factors for an appropriate balance in brain chemicals. This balance is necessary to promote a healthy mind and thus

<u>a healthy body. If you do activities, chronically knowingly or unknowingly, to rob yourself of dopamine, serotonin, noradrenaline and other chemicals – you become stressed, feel anxiety and remain depressed. You become vulnerable to addictions in order to get those chemicals replenished externally at the cost of your precious health. You indulge in smoking, alcohol, etc. Remember, you have only one body and one mind to smoothly sail through life; there is no replacement here.</u>

The responsive CEO, the reactive CEO & the executive –

The higher calculative and reasoning centre with higher thoughts is the responsive CEO and it is also the enforcement engine (this is the frontal lobe and pre-frontal cortex). We can enforce control over our body and mind even when they crave something from this centre. Like even we are starving, we do not snatch delicious food from the person eating beside us. Therefore, it can mobilize other brain centres to solve new problems, generate new thoughts and create a new neural net with repeated practice. It loves new things and new challenges more than anything. It loves happiness, motivation and the flow of dopamine. It establishes the state and work from the government in a continuous feedback loop. It works best when our brain is at alpha, gamma & theta.

On the other hand, the reactive CEO, the midbrain, is the emotional brain and our emergency response brain (i.e., amygdala and other vibrant centres). It's our relay centre. If we feel a negative emotion, it relays the power to the stress buttons for emergency and creates the required response. If we think positively and productively, it will keep the brain functioning at our responsive CEO's hands. This part of the brain must create long-term memory by attaching emotions and experiences to short-term memory. It produces proper emotional cues to our memory and function. It can also have extremely adverse and emergency reactions in our body (stress) if we visualize, think, or predict a negative situation or a gloomy future. The prediction happens from the data stored in the memories full of experiences and emotions. These memories and experiences are stored and then projected from our cerebellum (the hard disk and RAM) to our conscious and subconscious mind to predict the circumstances and the future outcomes. The cerebellum is the seat of our sub-conscious mind. These centres make us who we are and determine how we think in accordance to our association (place, person and time) and past experiences.

Another characteristic of the responsive CEO is discovered when a new task or challenge is in its hand. It starts creating new models to solve it and goes on correcting itself (only if the relay machine of emotion is not promoting the stress response). After it successfully creates a new neural net, it calls for the action, as and when required. Then the cerebellum, mid-brain and other parts of the brain execute the action as per the requirement. Once hard-wired, the activity becomes a very natural activity for us.

For example, remember, when we first learned to ride a bicycle or drive the car? It was amusing and exciting as we were learning. We were motivated. Once we completed the learning process, we did not feel anything anymore. We can now do those activities naturally, with no extra efforts. It does not produce any excitement or motivation anymore because it's hard-wired and the subconscious mind has taken over.

Our mind is like an Operating System

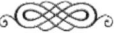

You already have the basic knowledge of how our brain may be working. It's clear from our earlier discussion that our brain is nothing but a highly advanced computing machine; it runs the operating system of our projected thoughts, beliefs and emotions. It computes billion of bytes of data per second and we only know a small amount of them.

The actively firing neural sets are what make us what we are today. It determines our personality as a whole. The way we think and the way we act are the results of these hard-wired neural nets. But at the same time, we should remember that these neural nets are modifiable by our thoughts, emotions and experiences in a feedback loop manner. Using our frontal lobe, we can push our body and mind to do new things; then, these new things become part of our automated learning with repeated activity. We already discussed this biological phenomenon in the earlier chapter. These projected thoughts and emotions from our sub-conscious mind create the interface of our operating system which is run by our brain, daily. These superficial and continuous thoughts randomly project thoughts, beliefs and ideas before getting our feedback on that thought process. As it goes on receiving affirmations, it goes on adjusting the thought process, the predictive model and the algorithm accordingly and continuously. That becomes the way we interact with the world around us and the manner in which we process the data.

Like any software system may require some updates from time to time, we also need to update some of these neural nets (thoughts and beliefs) from time to time, so that these serve us better in our life. The world around us is in a dynamic state; it's changing every second, but if we remain fixed in our lifetime, it may create a big problem. As the world is ever-changing, we need to upgrade our thoughts and beliefs, from time to time, to go beyond our difficulties and position ourselves with the altered circumstances. We can grow beyond and above our problems by creating a new state of mind. Thus, upgrading ourselves is not an option but is a necessity in today's world.

Now that we know the need for these upgrades is present, we should also gain some knowledge about how to upgrade our system? How to remove old, negative and unproductive neural nets? How to create new neural nets (thoughts and beliefs)? How to make them a part of our sub-conscious to automate them? For our convenience, we will call these neural nets the "app." We can uninstall the old app with errors and install a new app that serves us better. Thus, we can create an upgrade for our existing OS (Operating System).

The upgrade needs:-

How to uninstall the old app? In a given situation of life, you may find that an old habit or thought may seem not to be working anymore for our best. These thoughts then need change. But how we do that? For example, you have an app installed in your OS, "I am a busy person. I do not exercise." Now in your present life situation, your doctor already told you that you are having a cholesterol problem and borderline diabetes. Now you know that you need to start exercising regularly. It would be best if you also considered losing weight and thus, you may have a chance to lead a healthy life without any medication. You promised yourself that from that very day you would start your regular exercise. So, you get some knowledge from Google about the kind of exercise regime you should follow.

You have also surfed for days to find out the best rated TMT machine for your use. Now you would like some muscle in your body with a flat belly. You have always thought about that but could not do it. But this time you have also bought dumbbell, burble, ABB-exerciser and chest press table. You have also read some articles online about exercise and related activities. Now let's move the time to three months forward, where you find yourself not exercising again and gaining weight. Your purchased items are well-packed in a way that does not even produce a visual element anymore. From the healthy and muscular body that you hoped for in the future, you have shifted to your un-healthy diseased self again, in spite of yourself. Is this scenario known to you? The answer to this is probably "YES."

You know why is this happening? Because by telling yourself a declarative statement repeatedly, you have created a neural net, an app that runs a sub-conscious program of: "I am a busy person. I do not exercise." It fires now and then even without telling you. It projects thoughts, emotions and actions for you to avoid the situation of exercising successfully. And it does that without even notifying you. Remember, it is hard-wired in the past and is strengthened further with repeated feedback and declarations from our conscious mind.

The process to upgrade:

Now, the uninstallation of the unproductive app and simultaneously installing a productive app is required. The actions required as follows –

A. **Recognition:** Recognise clearly that not exercising is not helping you anymore. Practice to write journals as it's a great way to produce new thoughts and beliefs.

B. **Declaration:** Write down in the journal, "I am an athlete with great body fitness." Please, write it down ten times. Then read it or, if possible, write again and again every day, ten times in the morning and ten times before going to bed. Also, whenever you talk to yourself, declare, "I am an athlete." Declare this affirmative thought to yourself consciously again and again. Then the idea becomes hard-wired; the app gets installed. You will become the thought. You will start thinking, behaving, and acting according to your new statement, even unknowingly.

C. **Self-hypnosis and Visualisation:** Relax and visualise with your eyes closed. Relax and breathe. Practice visualization to imprint productive and affirmative thoughts on into your brain. So that these become your new habits.

The science behind it –

When you write in your journal, you are focused. You are also producing muscle memory by creating the thoughts and the experience of writing them, at the same time. When you repeatedly undergo the process, it accelerates the process of new neural net formation in accordance to the experience and the emotion that is in the journal. Keep doing it, and you will start noticing the change within 2 to 3 months.

When we repeatedly declare things to our mind, like, who we are, during the time that we are alert and awake, it creates a new neural net about "who we are?" and prunes down the neural net of "who we are not." The declarative memory with the repeated experience gradually becomes hard-wired in our brain.

When we visualize things vividly with strong emotions, we form memories. We already discussed that we could recreate any event in our mind without it happening, and it creates the same response in the brain and our body as if it were occurring in real-time.

Use visualization with the involvement of multiple senses and emotions to ensure that it is embedded into your memory. Thus, it automates those actions in your life that you wish for.

Move Into "The Zone Of Execution" - Use The Secrets Of Sports Psychology

The subconscious mind plays a crucial role in shaping our conscious activities. It might become a hindrance if we try to do something that we have never done before. Our subconscious mind's primary role is to keep us safe, and while doing so, it might make us stay in our comfort zone. Therefore, the first step towards making a massive change happen in our lives is to see the possibility of it happening. For example, if you have been in a comfortable job for many years but it does not resonate with your personality and passion, you need to believe that you can change it. In the beginning, you might apply to many relevant companies and might get rejected. Still, after being consistent, you will definitely get a reply from someone. This is what you need to make your subconscious mind understand. It needs to see that something always can happen.

In addition to that, it is essential to identify the resistances or impediments put forward by your subconscious mind because that affects your conscious activities significantly. Therefore, if you observe that something is holding you back from doing things that you love, you must ask yourself a few questions. Why is it that you feel better about procrastinating than actually finishing the task at hand? Why does achieving something that you want and have wanted for some time put you in a vulnerable position? After consciously addressing these questions, you will notice that the resistance from your subconscious mind will reduce. Little by little, you will feel more capable of doing things that you genuinely want to do.

The best thing is to focus on "WHAT" you want instead of obsessing about the "HOW." Once you start working towards what you want, you will start noticing new paths and opportunities. On the contrary, if you already start thinking about how something is impossible to achieve, you will never move in the right direction. So, even if you believe that people will deny your request, it is good to ask for it instead of deciding that it will be rejected without trying.

Hence, it is evident that our subconscious mind significantly shapes our conscious activities. By logically questioning and understanding the impediments put forward by our subconscious mind, we can substantially shape our intended actions.

Why Can't We Do Things Even If We Want To Do Them Consciously?

As already mentioned above, your subconscious mind is very powerful. According to psychologists, your subconscious mind handles 95% of your brainpower, making sure that you are comfortable physically and mentally. Its functions range from digesting food to breathing and eating, making memories and everything else that is necessary to survive. However, you must note that your subconscious mind is not creative at all. It can remember and store things that it witnesses but cannot find innovative or out-of-the-box solutions for your problems. Therefore, your mind becomes a hindrance, even if your conscious mind is willing to do something.

You can always take control of your subconscious mind and mould it in a way that it helps you do things, instead of becoming an impediment. Once you do that, you can be in control and achieve anything and everything you have always desired to have, but never dared to go for. The reason for it is simple; when both the conscious and the subconscious mind work together to achieve a common goal, your focus is high, and there are no obstacles to reaching your goals.

If you want to do something or achieve your goals consciously, but you feel something is stopping you, these are the many things that can help you break the barrier:

- **Get In Touch With Your Mind**

It may sound a little absurd, but getting in touch with your subconscious mind is an excellent technique to understand yourself and your inhibitions. You can do this by taking part in a simple meditation every day with no distractions. Even sitting quietly for 10 minutes a day can help you understand many things inside your subconscious mind. It will also help you strive for a balance between your conscious and unconscious mind and help them work towards a common goal.

- **Develop A Habit Of Writing**

Many psychologists have stated that writing is an excellent way of getting in touch with our subconscious mind. When we write something (a journal or a fictitious story), our subconscious mind plays a significant role in shaping the narrative. Hence, it helps reach out to some of our subconscious thoughts and emotions that we are not aware of consciously.

- **Visualization Technique**

Visualization is a great technique that can help your subconscious mind understand and process things. According to studies, people who visualize their goals are more likely to achieve them. It helps your subconscious mind believe that reaching your goal is possible because it looks more real when you visualize it. You can indulge in purposeful self-talk and create a helpful phrase for yourself. Using the techniques of visualization and positive self-talk can help you succeed in many sports as an athlete. It also positively impacts your recovery process after an injury. You can do it easily by slowly focusing on your breath and imagining yourself practicing the sport correctly. You can also relax your muscles and repeat the activity and steps mentally as per your coach's advice.

What Should We Do To Improve Our Execution?

It is essential to reprogram your subconscious self so that you can overwrite the damaging or limiting messages that it stores. Execution is everything in this regard, and you can either follow a few methods at a time or use all of them simultaneously to reap the maximum benefits. Whatever you choose, make sure that you focus your full attention on these methods to reprogram your subconscious rather than diluting your efforts or skipping ahead.

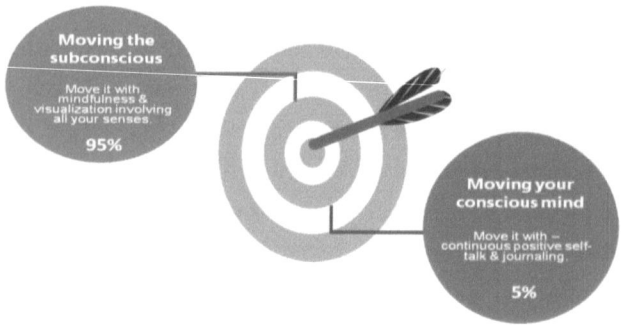

Figure 08: Showing importance of conscious as well as subconscious mind in action and execution

Failure to execute at will is a very big source of stress and anxiety. So, let us discuss few ways to improve execution:

- **Environmental Influences**

First and foremost, the environment has a significant influence on our subconscious mind. In this regard, it is crucial to remember that our subconscious mind always absorbs information, data and forms beliefs and draws conclusions based on all of this. Hence, if the environment you live in daily is loaded with strife and negativity, your mind will absorb some of the most hostile and harmful messages from its surroundings. Therefore, the first action that you must take right now is to limit all the negativity surrounding you. You must avoid watching the news and limit your time with people who negatively influence you. We should weed out such toxic people out of our lives. Also, you must seek positive information, as much as possible, by spending time with successful and positive people and watching and reading optimistic and happy things. Once you embrace this method, you will notice that, over time, your mind will absorb more encouraging messages, and you will be able to witness your true potential.

- **Affirmations**

If you want your mind to absorb some positive messages, you can also use the technique of affirmations. You can carry out this technique by following a few simple rules. To begin with, you must use all the affirmations in the present tense and word them positively. For instance, you can say things like, "I am successful and confident" instead of "I will be successful and confident." This is because the subconscious mind does not understand the future and only knows the present. Also, you must avoid using negatives as your subconscious does not understand them either. So, instead of saying, "I am a failure," you can try saying, "I am not a failure." In the same vein, it is also essential to feel your affirmations. So, if you say "I am wealthy," and you do not feel wealthy, the affirmation will amount to nothing as your subconscious mind will not believe it. Finally, you must keep repeating your affirmations as they won't work simply by enunciating them for a time or two. Keep reciting them throughout the day and make them a part of your routine.

- **Visualization and Hypnosis**

Studies have shown a positive correlation between external and internal imagery regarding performance in sports among athletes. Athletes who practice Taekwondo, use sensory experiences such as olfactory, kinaesthetic, visual, and auditory internally as a first-person and externally as a third person, which enhances the sport performance immensely. A sport like Taekwondo relies as much on physical as on mental skills.

By practicing some of these techniques, you can strike a balance between your conscious and subconscious mind. Once you achieve it, you will notice that you will be more synchronized towards achieving your goals, and there will be no obstacles. That is when you will see that you can do all the things you want to do consciously without barriers.

Hypnosis is another effective way of reprogramming your subconscious mind. Hypnotists work by making you talk in a more receptive and relaxed state and helping you deliver empowering and positive messages to your subconscious mind. You can also opt for self-hypnosis by using pre-recorded audio programs rather than a live session. It is even possible to record self-hypnosis CDs of your own to hear yourself reciting positive affirmations in a relaxed state.

As the Olympian gold medallist rightly said –

"I am a big believer of visualization. I run my races mentally, so that I feel even more prepared."

- **Persistent and Consistent Reinforcement**

It is essential to take heed of the fact that reprogramming your subconscious mind takes time and effort. It requires consistency, persistence and perseverance. You will not see any immediate changes in yourself. Only by being persistent in the positive messages that you deliver to your subconscious mind will you start reaping the benefits of these methods. Once the changes become more evident, it will be a huge confidence booster for you, and you will become motivated to work towards improving yourself. The right motivation is to know that these changes will be powerful, worth it, and lifelong, once you embrace these techniques and conquer your subconscious mind.

By following these few methods, you can retrain your subconscious mind into making you thrive and letting go of things that hold you back, such as procrastination and negativity.

Applying sports psychology to your daily life is an excellent way to move into the execution stage and conquer your subconscious mind. Sports psychology is essentially the study of how behaviour and thoughts influence athletes' performance and vice versa. This technique has proved to be useful in increasing motivation and enhancing the performance of athletes. This technique makes use of training and sports to help people improve their well-being and overall lives. Some ways that you can apply sports psychology in your daily lives to move into execution are:

Sports psychology deals with using athletics to manage your mind-set and get rid of negative emotions. Therefore, you can reap the most benefits by working on your deepest thoughts and making yourself better from the inside out. Working with a psychologist is a good idea as they are qualified experts who can help you understand yourself better. Some clinical reports even show that when sports teams and athletes work with psychologists, they enjoy improved emotional and mental health. Adopting these easy tools can go a long way in weeding out those deeply buried emotions and making your subconscious mind more in tune with your conscious self.

Only by following these simple sports psychology techniques can you get leverage over your subconscious mind and lead a more fulfilled and happier life.

Make stress your friend and ride it like a Sports Car.

In this chapter, you will learn to build the arsenal of resilience. Own the "arsenal of resilience" and form a friendship with stress. Stress is GOOD and necessary for life and action. "Stress" is the engine of our sports car (body-mind complex). Like a sports car, we should also have excellent steering, great brake and other safety tools alongside stress. It is not only the engine power which matters but also the other safety features, without which the rider may end up dead.

The stress is necessary for us to function. Stress hormones are highest in the morning when we wake up in the morning. When we take daily challenges in life, theses hormones reach their peak. We find our heart rate is racing, we are sweating and our pupils dilate. Our body is preparing ourselves to take action at that moment. These are necessary and without these, we are pretty much vegetation.

The problem happens when there is no brake into this acceleration. The problem occurs when we are always thinking about something, some nagging unproductive thoughts that are of no meaning or significance. Stress is necessary for us to perform at our best, but knowing how to run the stress with brakes and with all other safety measures is also essential in today's world. In today's business world, a single callous activity may lead to a disastrous result. So we need high speed and lots of stress hormones with proper balance and control. We need to automate these controls in your sub-conscious so that conscious effort need not be taken by ourselves every time everything happens. As I believe, "Chronic stress" kills (Vide chapter 1: Body in Chronic Stress), but acute stress is necessary.

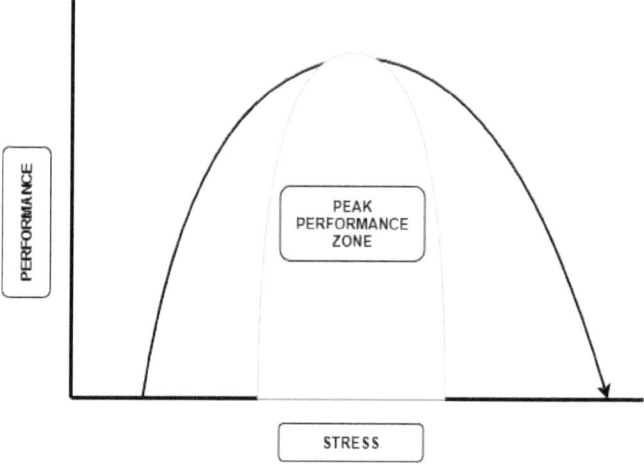

Figure 09: Showing the relationship between stress and performance.

The method to put brakes and safety into that engine will be discussed in this chapter. Do not sacrifice the engine itself. Stress is necessary for action just like the engine is necessary to run the car. But let's not waste oil and engine power on random power generation especially when it is not required. Use most of your energy to run the wheels.

Two factors are essential here for consideration —

1. Ability to FILTER the thoughts.

2. Ability to have an empty mind at will.

1. Ability to filter the thoughts— As you notice, ideas are often thrown at us by our wandering mind. Like we wear sunglasses to avoid unnecessary and excessive sunlight, wear the filters of your positive and productive thinking to avoid excess ideas.

2. Ability to have an empty mind as and when required— This is a muscle that a leader must develop; otherwise, a continuous loop of thoughts create unnecessary long-term stress, even in the absence of the stressor. These constant unproductive thoughts are either about a past adverse event or a future prediction of negative probability. Both of these are disturbing and produce chronic stress, leading to lesser productivity and damage to our health and well-being.

Stress, by all means, should be utilized for high performance, to reach and test one's limitation, to learn new things, and to do productive works. It deals with multiple areas as it's a big engine. But the knowledge of what oil (thoughts) to put inside the engine and how the brake (capacity to stop the thoughts at will) is become the most critical factors to consider, rather than driving the car itself.

Stress is our friend; it is the powerhouse of our life. It must be used properly for great results. It is necessary not to forget the other parts as you can't blame the engine behind the malfunctioning of a car. Remember, other significant factors determine the car's high performance and it safely reaching the destination; thus probably it malfunctioned because you did not install proper brakes or put the necessary oils inside it.

Where is the "BRAKE?" Why it is NOT working?

Simple, you are neither cleaning it nor doing the necessary maintenance. There's a cognitive difficulty due to lack of regular maintenance. It requires actualization and cleansing.

Let's discuss the "BRAKE." It's a muscle and so it needs the practice to develop. But once established it provides a higher safety with significant amount of stress. We need this cognitive function by our side and it requires daily maintenance.

Journaling –

Acknowledgment journaling– Write down three events of your life where you lost control over your thoughts. Surely, those thoughts persisted for days, consistently producing a state of irritation and lower productivity. It stayed even when you did not have anything to do about it. The thought persisted and created stress even when nothing was happening in front of you. Please write down your feelings about how you have lost your precious energy and focus over it and became a slave of your loop of thoughts.

Practice Stillness Of Non-judgmental Awareness– SNA Meditation

If you are unsure about the benefits of meditation, it is a must to know that not only does it help you mentally but it also assists you in physical health as well. Once you start practicing it, you will know how beneficial it is for your overall well-being. It improves our cognitive function, reduces stress-anxiety and depression, prevents heart attack, its related diseases and their complications, improves our decision-making abilities, happiness, executive capabilities– the list is pretty long.

We clean our body with soap and water daily. We clean our teeth when we brush daily. We clean our bowel almost daily. But what about listening and cleaning our minds of unnecessary and unproductive thoughts? How do you do that? Everyday our mind gives rise to many negative thoughts and ruminations which are not useful. We need to observe these thoughts non-judgmentally and see them passing by or release them, if necessary. We can focus on an important thought too. This is the process of meditation. Healthy lifestyle is incomplete without it. **Practice SNA MEDITATION.**

Meditation is the practice of thinking deeply or focusing one's mind for some time. While many forms of meditation exist, the main purpose of it is a feeling of inner peace and relaxation which can reduce anxiety and depression.

Depression continues to be a serious health issue among millions of people. It affects about 20% of adults, who are of 65 years of age and above.

Regular depression leads to higher risks of heart diseases and even death.

Researchers from Johns Hopkins University, in Baltimore, did analyse 19,000 meditation studies and 47 trials. Through their research and findings published in *JAMA* Internal Medicine on Monday, suggest that mindfulness in meditation does help to:

- manage psychological stresses like anxiety and depression

- manage pain
- prevent sleep issues
- prevent substance abuse
- prevent weight gain

With that in mind, let's take a look at the 12 ways meditation helps in reducing anxiety and depression:

- Meditation decreases activity in the brain's "Me Centre." According to a study carried out at Yale University, **mindfulness meditation reduces activity in the default mode network (DMN)**, the brain network which is responsible for self-referential thoughts and mind-wandering.

- It causes volume changes in key areas of the brain. A study suggests that mindfulness meditation may lead to **decreases in brain cell volume in the amygdala**, which is attributed to fear, anxiety, and stress.

- Helps the brain by **protecting the hippocampus**. Study has shown that people who meditated 30 minutes a day for eight weeks boosted the volume of grey matter in their hippocampus. Additionally, another research has shown that people with a smaller hippocampus are more prevalent to recurrent depression.

- Meditation can **alter reactions to stress and anxiety**. Meditation trains the brain to return to focus when emotions and negative thinking intrude upon it.

- Increases **imagination and creativity.** Meditation allows us to tap the deeper, wiser dimensions of our minds; the areas which tend to speak in whispers.

- It can **help with addiction**. Research has found that mindfulness training can help people recover from various types of addictions.

- It helps you to **reduce negative emotions** and gain a new perspective on stressful situations. According to Dr. Denninger, you tend to ignore the negative sensations of stress and anxiety when you meditate. Meditation can give you a sense of peace, balance and calm that's beneficial for both, your overall health and emotional well-being.

- Meditation can help you build skills to manage your stress and it **increases your self-awareness.**

- It **helps to switch from reactive fight-or-flight responses** to a more thoughtful mode that's crucial for balanced decision-making.

- Finally, research shows that meditation can **help to reduce cancer survivors' fear of the illness coming back.** While meditation is not used to treat diseases like breast cancer, its supportive care is designed to assist a person to deal with the stress that comes with cancer. According to a study done on June 2, 2017, at the American Society of Clinical Oncology (ASCO), the fear of recurrence of cancer was reduced significantly in 222 cancer survivors who had undergone a meditation intervention.

The simplest way to meditate -

The basic form of meditation that, if practised, can take you far and help you to clean your mind is **Stillness of Non-judgmental Awareness (SNA.).** In this meditative form you have to sit comfortably and close your eyes; avoid distractions and relax. Now all you have to do is just observe your breath. Your thoughts will come and go. Some thoughts may able to capture your attention and make you run behind it. If that happens, just bring your attention back to your breath. Do not judge yourself or any of your thoughts. It is just you, your breath and the stillness around you. The thoughts will come and go before your non-judgmental awareness. This is how you can achieve **SNA**. – the simplest form of meditation.

Practice journaling with open-eyed mindfulness. Countdown from 5 to 1 and write the letter "A" and look at it for 5 seconds without chasing or judging your thoughts. Make an increment of 5 seconds every week, when you look at the letter. Failure is good, but do not bother yourself with judgments. Practice this twice, daily. Within three months, you will be the master of "the stillness of non-judgmental awareness" (SNA). You will experience a stillness where neither are your thoughts hijacking you nor arechasing any ideas. Here you are an observer; an observer who is merely observing his breathing.

The stillness is "beautiful," and non-judgmental awareness is the "least biased intelligence."

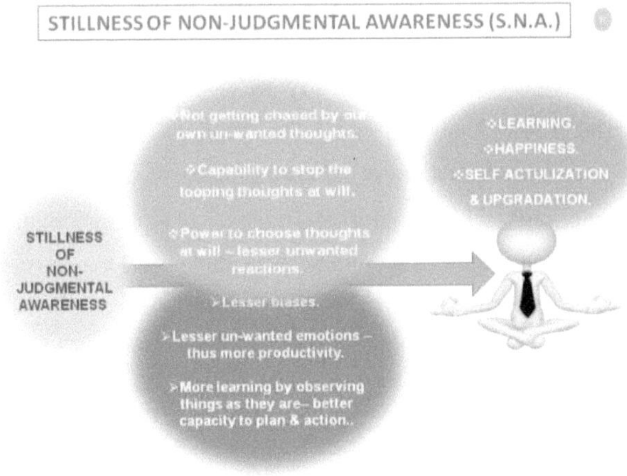

STILLNESS OF NON-JUDGMENTAL AWARENESS (S.N.A.)

- Not getting chased by our own un-wanted thoughts.
- Capability to stop the looping thoughts at will.
- Power to choose thoughts at will – lesser unwanted reactions.
- Lesser biases.
- Lesser un-wanted emotions – thus more productivity.
- More learning by observing things as they are – better capacity to plan & action.

STILLNESS OF NON-JUDGMENTAL AWARENESS

- LEARNING.
- HAPPINESS.
- SELF ACTULIZATION & UPGRADATION.

Figure 10: Showing the importance of meditation (Stillness of Non-judgmental Awareness) in terms of our cognitive improvements.

Write down the following benefits of SNA in your journal-

1. A minute of SNA is the muscle power to stop and discard negative and unproductive thoughts at will.

2. A minute of SNA is a "space" where you can write many new things throughout the day.

3. A minute of SNA is the window where new ideas flow into you.

Mindfulness- Sit comfortably. Close your eyes. Relax and count from 5 to 1. Breathe. Distribute gratitude to your past. Distribute gratitude to the universe. Observe your breath.

Count your breath down from 5 to 1 and be the master of the precious "SNA" with a closed eye. The more you practice, the more power you will hold. Try to develop at least twelve breaths SNA. Learn to enjoy the "stillness" and praise the non-judgmental awareness as you achieve it. Thus you will have the capacity to develop more power to stop the engine as and when necessary. The more power the engine can save, the more it can re-direct energy to useful work.

The S.T.O.P.
(Self-talk Optimizer Protocol)

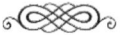

"Don't be a VICTIM of the negative talk, remember, YOU are listening." – Bob Proctor

Did you notice that a voice is always with you? It talks many times completely unprovoked or without conscious effort from you. It gives you the immediate impressions of events, and mostly if untrained, the voice speaks of negative consequences and negatively about the time, the place, and the person. It also tells you about some very twisted adverse outcomes sometimes, a distant probability which even you do not believe. It interacts with you in a feedback loop manner. The more you nod at its negative output, the more it becomes active. It can spiral down or spiral up things at infinite depths or infinite heights, respectively. It's a great weapon gifted to us by nature. We should use it for our productivity. But like all weapons, it can be used to produce a negative and unproductive mind-set.

We may, at times, need to apply the S.T.O.P (the Self Talk optimization protocols) in our lives. Continuous negative self-talk, about our own selves, produces low self-esteem. Constant negative self-talk about others and the world creates a depressed mood and robs us of the chemicals of happiness and motivation.

Wherefrom does it come? It's the projection from our sub-conscious mind. These are the immediate or superficial thoughts that get generated continuously by our Bayesian brain. It helps us analyse things to get predictive feedback from our experience before sensing and verifying items with reasons derived from the frontal lobe of our brain. If an event presses our emergency button, it bypasses the frontal lobe. It enters our emotional centre to produce an immediate reaction to our body-mind and the external world.

It can be trained for high performance "productive activity" and tuned down to produce low performance "unproductive activity." It can create a field of explosives for a long time and cause a disproportionate explosion in unexpected circumstances.

The short story

Kumar said, "Brother, can you come to our anniversary next week? It will be my great pleasure if you came with your family? Please." Kumar requested his younger brother, Manu, to attend the anniversary programme of Kumar and Kankana after a long time. They have a 10-year-old son name Knish. They live in Kolkata. Manu went to work in Ireland for a software company and returned to Delhi again, after ten years, as his company started operating in India. Manu got married there with Shree. They have a 4-year-old beautiful baby daughter name Boni. Manu replied with some neutral state of mind, "Let's see what I can do." "Please come; we all will feel good. Apart from that, please come and talk to our father too. He would also like to see you. You know, after our mother's death, he always took care of us. He was both our father and our mother. Please come."

Now the conversation ends here. But now, the conversation starts from within and inside Kumar, it goes something like this, "I know Manu is not going to attend our anniversary. Kankana was right. He never attends family ceremonies. On top of that, he probably still holds the grudge about his marriage to Shree. He did not even invite our father for a blessing. He still holds on to the hatred about how father used to love me more and scolded him in the past. He does not take responsibility of our father. Even if he attends any ceremony, he never talks to anyone properly. Also, if he talks to anybody, he starts judging them and hurting them as

well. He is a family embarrassment in the gatherings." In this manner the

talk goes on, in the day-time and even at night. Sometimes these thoughts also get a nod from Kankana, to say the absolute truth and there is no other way around it.

Now let's examine the thoughts inside Manu —"It's just a show-off call. I know that he never wants me around. My father, too, was always biased to Kumar. Father always praised Kumar, but never me. If my mother had been alive, things would have been different. The universe has always conspired against me from childhood. I always got the worst things in life. I did not get a good rank in the Joint Entrance, so my father spent money to make me an engineer in a private engineering college. Kumar poked me about that so many times.

Oh my GOD! I can't believe I will go to that

place . . ." and so on it goes.

This continues for days and nights. Now, Shree is persisting in going to this programme because she never met Manu's family. Now despite not wanting to go to the programme, Manu agreed to attend for Shree.

At the programme, Kumar meets Manu and Shree. Kumar smiled and greeted, but Manu neither noticed it nor welcomed Kumar properly. They just exchanged some words and that was it. Shree also started to feel Manu behaving weirdly. Manu simply greeted his father, but forgot to ask about his ongoing diabetes and blood pressure treatment or express how much he is missing his father. Manu only spent his whole time sitting on a chair without chit-chatting with his brother or other relatives. Kumar gets the cue that his brother has not changed and Manu keeps his belief about his brother as before. The family meeting was a complete failure because of the other ongoing thoughts.

On the way back, Shree asked Manu how the party was. Manu suddenly burst with the anger, "Don't you know? Why are you asking? It was your plan to make this bullshit trip." Shree replied, "Listen! They are your family. Do not shout at me for them. It's your problem and your brother's problem. Don't take your anger out on me,"

The conversation that goes on, now, is full of anger and despair for days. Manu consider that the whole trip was a "bad idea," and he promises himself that he will not visit his family again under any circumstance.

The Story Ends- What has happened?

Frankly, nothing extraordinary has happened. It could've been a great family meeting as whatever happened has happened in the mind of both brothers. They both predicted the family programme as per their old memories and successfully created the situation at par with their prediction. This is an endless loop. Until someone does something very extraordinary, it will remain the same. Even if Manu never visits his family, he will have a nagging thought about the event for months. You see how our negative talk can successfully rob us of our family events and create a mental storm and family quarrel even when nothing has happened. The reaction to the game was that Manu will never visit is family; this reaction is out of proportion.

We can make the same event happen to ourselves, our profession, and our organizations daily; the out of proportion negative outcome to an ordinary event. "There were many terrible things in my life, and most of them never happened." - Michel de Montaigne, philosopher of the French Renaissance.

Let's analyse the science behind the story: By continuously running the old memories in their brain, both brothers have predicted an adverse event. They played the same negative outcome of the forthcoming programme. They convinced themselves of this through continuous visualization. They programmed their subconscious mind so well that they overlooked many brighter facts of the story. The elder brother took care to call his younger brother after such a long time, and he requested many a time for his younger brother to come. Their father misses his younger son too. The father also spent a lot of money on his younger son's career, and the father always took care of them. The younger brother also received an excellent welcome upon arrival. But as both brothers pictured so many negative thoughts and repeatedly played them in their brain, they thought the only future, awaiting them, is just the repetition of the past itself. The younger brother behaved accordingly; the elder brother readily accepted the negative outcome as an expected fact. We cannot produce positive results with a negative mind-set. "Insanity: doing the same thing over and over again and expecting a different result."- Albert Einstein.

That's why the most unbiased observer here, Shree, could not understand what happened there. Most of it has happened inside the head of the two brothers. Nobody thought or visualized any of this and thus they acted differently and positively. Therefore, a family meeting, that could have been a memorable and beautiful event, was converted into a complete embarrassment without provoking the ceremony itself.

There are more examples

Do you know a person who is living in the realm of constant irritation? You can ask him anything, but you will always get an answer of irritation. He would still burst into unnecessary and out of proportion anger, in many events. He neither likes himself nor anybody in this world. If you know him, you should know he is a product of constant negative self-talk.

Do you know a person who believes that he could not be successful in anything in life? He believes that everything that he would do will fail. So he recreates those in reality and gives examples of his failures to everyone. If you know him, you should know he is a product of constant negative self-talk.

Do you know a person with enough wealth, achieved many things in life, but is unable to be happy and a little satisfied in his daily life? He is always telling himself that he did not accomplish enough. He is continuously telling himself about the negativity of his present circumstances. If you know him, you should know he is a product of constant negative self-talk.

We may think that when we are alone and nobody is listening, we can talk however we want to ourselves and that it doesn't matter. But you should know, at this point, that it does matter the most. When you tell negative things to you about yourself or another place, person or event, you create a new thought process; you create a new predictive algorithm in your subconscious mind, creating a gloomy mood for yourself. What else could be more harmful than this self-destructive habit? Take care of your self-talk. Remember: you become your self-talk.

So, what would be the solution?

Remember, every journey to change or upgrade ourselves starts with the realization in our mind that something needs to change. The solutions are as follows:

Be aware - If you become aware of your self-talk and train it to tell you productive things and the positive things, it will get taught. It's your monkey and you are the master. With repetition, it will get trained and serve you better.

Write Journals — You also should write journals about your unproductive and negative thoughts daily. You can write in your journal why those thoughts are not serving you any good at present and will not serve you any good in the future. You should then declare that this thought doesn't belong to you and release your mind's idea. After this is done, put some positive thoughts in that place.

Use visualization and mindfulness meditation –Sit comfortably, breath in a regular pattern and relax yourself completely. Free yourself of your negative self-talk.

Optimize your self-talk before you go out to do something. If you are bombarding your mind with negative self-talk, you cannot do positive things in your life.

Flexibility is the KEY

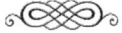

> "A human being is a part of the whole called by us universe, a part limited in time and space. He experiences himself, his thoughts and feeling as something separated from the rest, a kind of optical delusion of his consciousness. This delusion is a kind of prison for us, restricting us to our personal desires and to affection for a few persons nearest to us. Our task must be to free ourselves from this prison by widening our circle of compassion to embrace all living creatures and the whole of nature in its beauty."
>
> *-Albert Einstein*

Before a person goes out there, into the world, and starts leading his professional and personal life, he should understand how the world is, in a very objective manner. Without understanding how the world is, often, the leader may fall into the trap of his absolute considerations. The following are the characteristics of the world.

R.P.M. World Point of View- (Relative, Probabilistic and Multifactorial)

A. Understanding that this is a relative world- We must realize that this is a relative world.

Our thoughts, opinions and beliefs are relative in nature. Something true for us may not be right for another person. Some of our limitations and our outlook of the world may not be true for others.

Our thoughts and beliefs were shaped by our past experiences, combined with our emotions.

The past experiences are unique to people and their emotional affect with those experiences is also different.

Please acknowledge the relativity of your thoughts and beliefs before you go outside the world to manage others.

We also need to acknowledge that more counter beliefs are incorporated while making a decision; the more we recognize the relativity of a decision, the better decision we take.

The more we respect others' individuality and uniqueness, and our own thoughts' relativity, the less stressful our lives would become.

B. Understanding that the outcomes are probabilistic- The outcome of our actions is probabilistic. No matter how absolute we think the outcome would be, it, by all means, is probabilistic. The strength always has an in-built weakness. The opportunities always have inbuilt threats and vice-versa. Remembering this while considering your ideas or your business' strength and opportunities is vital. Remember, it's a matter of probability that your actions will produce the desired results, that your requests or orders will be executed, or that an alternate probability always exists. Remember, there is a factor in the known factor which is referred to as "unknown." Expect the best, take actions for the best, but never forget that things do not happen in life for you or targeting particularly YOU. These are not about YOU; these happen with a probability in a given scenario and probability does not need to favour you always. The sense of probability will reduce your business stress by at least half.

C. Understanding the involvement of multiple factors deciding an outcome – We need to remember that an outcome always has various positive as well as negative factors. These factors shape the way for the outcome. In any scenario, these factors must be remembered. These provide a more significant source of flexibility to any situation. Remember, if you consider only one aspect or one person to be responsible for something, that consideration should be reviewed. It will give you a better detailing of the situation. The more factors that you have in your hands for modification, the better you can perform.

Power of Query-

Understanding the power of self-control and the power of query: Query is a powerful tool which helps us keep our reactions in check. It helps us get information from others to build our analysis for a situation. If we express our opinions directly to our team, we may miss out on information. That may not be very objective among so many things, including our emotions. Almost always, it is biased negatively. This is where the blame game starts. In these situations, we are practically headed towards a heated discussion. The situation does not solve the problem rather it creates more problems on top of already existing ones. It is ideal to follow power of query for any given situation and move your team towards a productive direction.

Here are the emotional barriers to query:

After a situation, or say a challenge, arises immediately there appears the "FIRST TRAP" which is emotional hijacking. We get hijacked by our immediate negative emotions into a conclusion without any detailed analysis. Be self-aware that immediately after something happens you become your thoughts. In-spite of observing the thoughts in a non-judgmental way and then choosing the most productive one, we become our immediate thoughts more often than not. Be aware that the FIRST RISK is inside you, and that you can control it. Always be biased about the fact that your immediate conclusions may not be the fact they are your relative opinions about a multifactorial outcome. Hold on to yourself, observe your thoughts and be non-judgmental when you are at it. Calm down and observe your breath for a minute or so.

After you have learned well about how to overcome the "FIRST TRAP," the most incredible tool to master is the "power of query." Ask someone something and then observe him with non-judgmental awareness. It will give you a lot of information about things of which you had no idea earlier. You will start noticing both – "told" and "un-told" stories. Utilise the query power as a useful tool and then use the "power of query" to the situation with an open mind.

1. Power of "What"

Be non-judgmental. Observe your breath while counting from 5 to 1. Slow down your breathing to 8 to 10 breaths per minute. Always begin with the person involved with the query of "WHAT"– let him narrate the story for you. Observe his facial expressions, attitudes and realize the untold part of the story while listening to the "WHAT." Be mindful and focused at this point. Be non-judgmental in the moment.

2. Power of "why"

If you want to know the productive root cause of someone's emotions or expressions, the question to ask is "why." You can always ask a series of WHY at least five to a maximum of six. The first two "WHYs" have the power to exclude the most futile information. The next two, "WHYs," with proper moderation, can almost always give you the adequate root cause. Be aware of diversions, be mindful, be in the present and observe the person in front of you for every detail. Maintain eye contact and keep a watch out for un-told stories.

3. Power of "When"

> It is the most critical part of our day. There are many stories which people are telling us for our "to-do" list.

Know your step 1 - Be aware to always ask when. Just have a look into your resources and rely on your skill, if your resources and abilities can't match the "to-do" right now. In that case, note down in your journal and assign it a time when you can think about it. If it is urgent, consider how you can re-arrange your resources and your skill to match the challenge. If you still can't manage it, arrange for people with the resources and the skills to meet challenges.

If those "to-dos" are productive for you, decide upon how you can match your skills and resources to meet the short-term to medium-term challenges. Always upgrade yourself for the long-term to meet your long-term challenges. The long-term up-gradation plan is a must-have.

Avoiding the "FIRST TRAP" and having the "ABILITY TO LISTEN TO OTHERS MINDFULLY" are the keys to success in business and life. Try to listen what is not told. Try to see what is not shown. A non-judgmental focused presence can show you many things that you would have otherwise missed. Own this power in order to sail through your daily challenges with your team members.

Again, you can do so with the help of journaling. First, prepare the journal, then write it yourself and finally read for at least 60 days to start getting results. Move your sub-conscious with mindfulness and visualization to automate these inside your brain. Let's begin.

Install the art inside your sub-conscious-

1. Journaling – Be aware of how many times, throughout the day, you are propelled by your absolute thoughts and thereby disregard the relative world concept. Be aware how many times you believed that X is only caused by Y, there you disregarded the underlying multiple factors which affect an outcome. Be aware how many times you considered that an intended outcome has 100% probability if you do X.

   Be aware and do the journaling about these absolute and rigid thoughts of yours. It will be more prudent and less stressful if you live your life with more flexibility by considering that the world and your thoughts are relative, the outcomes are multifactorial and the intended future is probabilistic.

Write down your flexible thoughts by replacing the absolute one.

2. Mindfulness – Relax and achieve a deep meditative state (i.e. self-hypnosis), as we have discussed earlier. Meditate on: "the world and my thoughts are relative; my present-day outcomes are multifactorial; and my intended future is probabilistic. I do thank the universe to collapse the threads of probability in my favour. I do thank everyone for both the good and the bad to shape my path."

Rule The Reactions

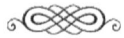

> "**Between stimulus & response, there is a space. In that space is our power to choose our response. In our response lies our growth & our freedom.**"

VIKTOR FRANKL

Our reactions are nothing but the hijacked state of our mind. In this state, our long term and productive options are not available to us.

Sometimes when an event occurs, our immediate response and the things that we say "at the moment" happen involuntarily and without any control. To a reasonable extent, this is true. How many times have we used inappropriate and cuss words to justify our anger? How many times have we reacted without thinking? And how many times have we commented, in real life or on social media, on things that needed more understanding?

When an event occurs in the world outside, then almost immediately a reaction occurs inside our head. Our sensory system perceives it with inputs from our survival mode, which mostly uses negative experiences of our past, causing our negative emotions to get attached to it. Before we decide, we often act within a fraction of second.

We need to develop a mental faculty, a way of handing stimulus so that we do not get hijacked by our negative and survival thoughts every now and then, even in a non-emergency situation, like sitting in our office. Then we can build a long-term productive decision which makes sense. In the business world, preventing unwanted reactions is an essential functional requirement in our everyday life.

While the immediate response is suitable for an emergency, it may prove inappropriate while sitting in our office, making business decisions or while sitting with our family and friends and building relationships for the long term.

It might sound like what we say is always an immediate reaction, and there is barely anything we can do about it. But it is time we understand that it does not have to be that way. We need to install a space between the stimulus and response, and only then will we be able to decide how we should react in a given situation.

If we install a space between the stimulus and response, we can keep our immediate predictive thoughts to be positive and the direct emotions motivated; no matter what, the emotional part of our action remains under the guidance of the "CEO" of our brain (known as the pre-frontal cortex). The CEO of the mind can only perform analysis and do the creative work for us. A whole ocean of options opens up.

We can choose what we want to say or how we want to react in a situation; that is now up to us, and not up to the event or the person. The stimulus here need not necessarily determine our action leading to long-term consequences.

In this space, between our stimulus and our response, we can decide to remain productive.

Why is it essential to install the space?

We have already spoken about how ideas get positively affected the moment we decide to pause and reason. It is time to understand the psychology behind it. When we receive a stimulus to react, our immediate thoughts and emotions are animalistic due to our negative biases. When we activate the survival part of our brain (the amygdala), we only have the four F's ("flight," "fright," "fight," & "fornicate"). The negative biases (immediate thoughts and emotions) thus activate the survival part of the brain.

But in between any stimulus if we keep our immediate thoughts and emotions positive, then the animal or survival part of the brain does not get activated now and then. If the CEO of the brain (the pre-frontal cortex) remains on our side, then our creative and lateral thinking stays with us.

It is essential to understand how this works. Our animal instincts are sudden. The decisions that we take in such moments are often taken to protect ourselves. Emotions like "fear," "fight," or "flight" are often animalistic in nature. We require these emotions in acute emergencies only while in other situations, rational decision-making is required more. These rational decisions come from the CEO of our brain. It only gets into the action if our immediate thoughts and emotions are positive upon receiving a stimulus. Then the stimulus enters into the CEO of our brain, and it is only then that we can make creative decisions that involve some analysis.

If possible, sleep on an idea or problem. When we sleep soundly, our brain creates new synapses and processes the information in a more in-depth manner in order to give a better decision as the output.

The CEO of the brain works better with calmness, self-confidence and positive and secure thoughts. In 3F mode, it's just the animal brain that works mindlessly and that is mostly unproductive in business.

Thus, to become a "responsive being" again, two major factors need to be considered: 1. FACTOR A – The "CONFIDENT and SECURE SELF" and 2. FACTOR B – Capacity to filter out negative thoughts and emotions.

Become the CONFIDENT and SECURE SELF

Here, the "POSITIVE self-talk" becomes very important. Here's an example of positive self-talk to instil confidence: "I have already overcome so many obstacles in my life, and I will overcome anything. I can and I will. "

The secure self-talk is the state of being where you believe that the universe is not coming to destroy you, instead, it wants you to flourish. Here you consider the world as your friend and that it is conspiring for your good. "The universe itself secures me; the challenges are just testing me to become better. These are shaping me in a good way. I can always overcome even the worst situation."

Continue this positive self-talk. Write down these in your journals and do not allow the opposite to enter your mind. Do not chase the different thoughts, and do not judge. Simply look at things as they are and discard them at will from your account.

Install the space and rule the reactions –

How to manage our reactions?

List the five most common scenarios where you generally lose your composure. You can also think about your past events as an example of such situations. Describe your immediate thoughts and emotions that arise from within. Be non-judgmental to yourself. Just do descriptive journaling. Write down how you would avoid being hijacked by your negative thoughts and emotions. Concentrate on your breath, slow down your breathing, and then observe the thoughts passing by like clouds in the sky. If you cannot calm yourself down, ask yourself to do so, and leave the place for an interval. If not, try not to give any critical output; silence is a better option.

Training your sub-conscious –

Always remember to move your sub-conscious and install important thoughts inside your brain with repeated practice. As we mentioned earlier, to automate thoughts inside our minds, we need to do careful journaling and mindfulness with visualization.

1. Journaling– Write down how many times a day you have entered into the 3F mode in a secure office due to your negative biases. Write down what you would do the next time that such a situation arises. Write down that with every stimulus you will keep your superficial thoughts and emotions positive so that your creative thinking stays with you.

2. Be mindful and visualize– Be aware that as you go through your day or business meetings, how many

times are you entering into the animal mode swiftly due to a stimulus? How many times could you have been more creative? Be aware. Do not pass judgment on yourself, but be mindful. Discard your 3F self at will, and keep your creative and lateral thinking part by your side.

Mind Your Productive Categories

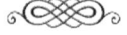

> "The way to get started is to quit talking
>
> and begin doing."
>
> -*Walt Disney.*

Most workplaces talk about productivity these days and to better understand productive categories better, we must first understand what the term "productive" actually means.

"Productivity"

"Productivity," in itself, means something useful. But then again, useful is exceptionally subjective. For example, a regular watch for a blind person is a useless object; it does not have any value even if it is a diamond-studded Rolex. So, a better term would be any work or issue that holds meaning to the person doing it.

Throughout the day, we often ponder upon things that are either unrelated to us or hold very little meaning in our lives. While doing so, we categorize them as "good" or "bad," "superior" or "inferior," and "black" or "white."

For example, Rohit reads about a business tycoon's money-laundering case and how his booming empire has now come to ruins. Throughout the day, Rohit thinks about how evil the person is and how much money he has stolen from people. Despite not being even remotely related to the case, or the person, or the business, Rohit's loss of productivity can be directly tied with these thoughts.

It is our inherent nature to judge and create categories for every issue that we come across. It could also be about events and people or almost any other thing. While judging is terrible in itself, not creating categories is even worse, because then it leaves little room for rational thinking. Imagine working on a project and continuously thinking about the person who broke in the signal when you were going for work?

Unproductive thoughts create unnecessary negative ruminations, which cause the brain to fog at the end of the day. The categories that we commonly develop, as a result of such unproductive thoughts, are immediate and thus impractical. A phenomenon from history that may seem "bad" when it happened may pave the way to become something "good" at other times and vice-versa. Such thoughts are always associated with politicians, film stars, and famous personalities. When their decisions do not appeal to us, we immediately conclude that they are bad people. However, when the same personality does something noteworthy or something which we find reasonable, our perception of that person changes.

In the infinite realm, there is nothing such as the ultimate good or the ultimate bad. In the previous chapter, we saw how absolutely destructive thoughts can be and why we must not give extreme conclusions, especially when it concerns people. These thoughts are nothing but the ruminations of our mind and don't do anything good for us. But it does make us feel exhausted at the day's end, even though we have not done much work. Thinking requires energy, and in some cases, it is equivalent to physical workout. So overthinking is unnecessary physical exertion that causes fatigue in our bodies.

We must always try to distance ourselves from any thought that arises in our mind, which either has a tiny probability of affecting us or does not demand any action. Such thoughts are useless and unproductive, and so we must be careful.

Therefore, categorizing thoughts is one of the best ways of improving productivity. It will help us manage our thoughts better and allow us to define what serves our purpose and what doesn't. It's fair to think about unprivileged people, but only when you want to contribute something towards helping them. If you are working on building a robotic arm that operates on the human body and is preoccupied with hungry people in Syria, then you are bound to become unproductive. Categorize your thoughts and think about poor people when you are not working on the robot.

The rumination on such unproductive categories and thoughts must be avoided for our own good. In the above example, we can see how mixing one thought with another can affect our productivity. We live in a world of distractions, and with the rise of smartphones and tablets, it has become easy for us to ponder upon a thought that has nothing to do with our work. It can be the funny video of a cat, or a horrific accident, or a cop chasing a thief for three miles; the distractions are limitless, so some companies have a strict policy of not using smartphones or other such devices at work.

But we must remember that it is not really about the device but rather about the way we think. When we get distracted by external objects, we allow that thing to enter the space we have created for our work.

Instead, we should be possessed by thoughts that demand our problem-solving skills and our action by executing the productive ideas. This is a careful approach to abundant living, and it should be followed by anyone who wants a far better yield or result. If you are a business owner, then think only about your business during work hours. If you are an artist, then think about improving your art when you are working. By categorizing correctly, you ensure that your energy levels are high and your level of brain fatigue is low. This attitude also keeps us motivated to do positive and productive things in life.

The science behind productive thoughts–

The most advanced part of our brain, also known as the pre-frontal cortex, likes to solve the problems. It malfunctions with self-conclusive categories, they are neither problems nor do they evoke any effort to create solutions. These categories of "good," "bad," "superior," "inferior," "black" and "white" give rise to ruminating and unproductive thoughts. It doesn't do any good for anyone. These do not bring our pre-frontal cortex, the CEO of the brain, into play. Thus, it prevents the motivating and mood-stabilizing chemicals in the brain (dopamine, serotonin, anandamide, etc.). Motivation and stable mood is necessary for us to "focus" on the present and execute productive actions. To bring our CEO of the brain to work, we need to become mindful of unproductive, self-conclusive and ruminating thoughts. We should start producing thoughts like what we can do about the information that we just received or if we cannot do anything about it. We should discard the ruminations at will. If we can do something about it, the thinking should be "when?" and "how?" These are problem-solving thoughts. These thoughts along with the belief that "I can solve a problem," motivates us to rise to the challenges in life. It stops the wandering of the brain and promotes focused work. It keeps us motivated and happy now. Remember, only after we believe that something can happen only then does the probability of happening occur. If we do not believe that a solution is possible, then probability of the solution is zero.

Manage Your FOCUS

The un-divided attention that we give while we socialize, talk, work, or cuddle reveal more than what we know. The focus on the present will tell you more than you are getting told. If you focus on the underlying message then things will become clearer to you. You will realize that there are things that matter to us, as humans, which we cannot see with our naked eye. You will listen and perceive more than that is being conveyed.

Focus is a very useful but finite currency. Spend with care.

This is called mindful living. Notice your breathing at the times when you are working. Regular breathing of 10 to 16 breaths per minute is good while focusing on a task. Your focused activity will be exhausted every 90 to 120 minutes; it is then time to take a break.

After 6 to 8 such focused activities your brain needs to recover and form new connections which happens when you recover or sleep for at least 7 hours a day. Your synapses are exhausted of the brain chemicals after repeated focused activities.

Multi-tasking is not possible when the activity is a new one and requires your analytical engine to be completely into that moment. Your brain has only one analytical engine. Consciously, it can work out one problem at any one point of time. You can do two tasks simultaneously only if both deal with the exact repetition of your expertise. Be conscious or you will miss the newer developments.

You will need to relax then for half an hour (that will not come from Facebook or WhatsApp or watching TV or negative criticism or ruminating negatively or indulging in unproductive thoughts about past and future).

Instead, the relaxation should come from exposure to sunlight for a minimum of 15 minutes, water intake of 500 ml, listening to music with eyes closed, may be some kind of dance or body movements, listening to comedy shows or short stories, an afternoon nap of 30 minutes, socializing with people you like and if possible "in person", exercising in the afternoon, being mindful about your breathing, practicing gratitude, positive visualization and positively talking about the self. At least two of the activities can be done in combinations to relax the mind and body and replenish the energy for focus.

These promote dopamine in brain and make you happier and stay more in the present. You need lesser addictions. When you don't follow such activities, you are putting yourself under great stress and it results in a lack of focus. Researchers have noticed a drop in concentration when too many activities are handled at the same time. Mood changes and people become more cringy, angry, and irritated after a certain point of time.

FOCUS is very important in life and those who lack focus can often miss out on opportunities, or on real human connections. It does not always mean a goal or a place that you are trying to reach. It means giving time and energy to things that should matter, things that are real and things that are important to us. FOCUS is an indispensable attribute that can allow you to become the best version of yourself. It can lead you to the pinnacles of success or it can bring you down; this will depend on how you use focus as a personal tool.

Know Your "Step 1"

There are a lot of things we decide for ourselves to do, but here is the catch, what we can do right now? What should be the productive "STEP 1?" To find out the productive action for a thought/ plan, two factors should be strongly considered –

1. The thoughts/ actions that we are considering should be productive for us; productive means it would make some changes in our lives towards a positive direction.

2. Availability of SKILL/ RESOURCES right NOW– If the skill and resources required for step 1 is NOT available to you right now, it straightforwardly states that it can't be done right now. So what we considered to be STEP 1 cannot be it.

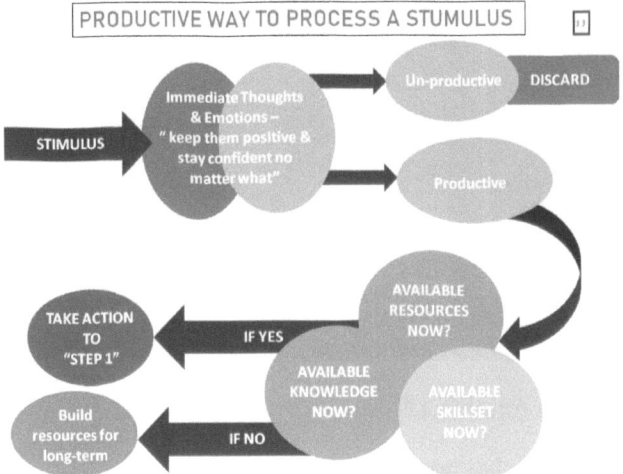

Now based on these factors, actions can be categorized as follows—

a. 1 & 2 both are present at NOW– Then that is "the STEP 1" and the next step is to start execution.

b. 1 & 2 both are absent– Discard the thought/ action at will, and continue the. search for " step 1".

c. 1 is high but 2 is low– These can be planned for the future as the skill and resources can be built over time. So start the planning process.

d. 1 is low but 2 is high – So basically there is a considerable scope of improvements to the quality of the thought and action. We should train our mind to talk of productive and positive things only.

Be aware about your step 1 and also learn to assign time to execute the same.

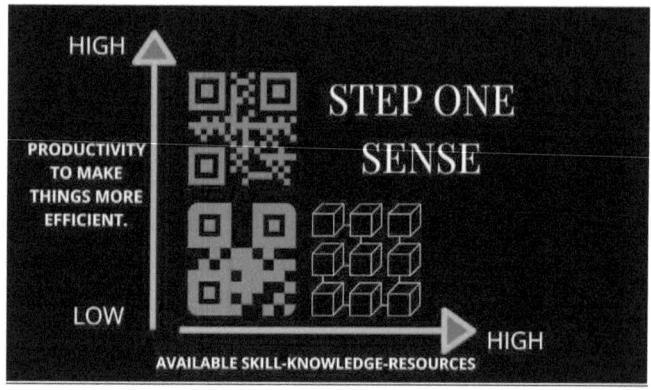

Manage Your FOCUS

"FOCUS" has two major attributes—

FACTOR A— State of motivation to execute "STEP 1," and

FACTOR B— Capability to manage distractions.

Following are the categories—

1. A & B both are high— this produces an intense capacity to "FOCUS".

2. A & B both are low— FOCUS is not possible.

3. A is high but B is low— Here, the person can focus but there will be disruptions.

4. A is low but B is high— Often focus is on unproductive things and the inability to find "STEP 1" leads to distractions and disruptions of the focus.

**Remember these are temporary and relative quadrants. You can acknowledge, act and change the quadrants at will. That's how change happens. That's the purpose of building the quadrants, to let you know where you are standing now and what actions will bring the growth and change; what would be required to improve and at what state of being.

So, let's begin the discussion.

a. Managing focus –

1. Manage your distractions– Whenever you are planning to start a work or you are scheduled for doing a project, manage you distractions carefully.

What will you do to the internet and notifications? You better turn it off, if it is not immediately necessary for your work and if the internet is necessary then open an account solely for work in your operating system; an account where you can only work.

What will you do to your phone notifications? – You better keep your phone in flight mode. If not possible put in silent mode and keep it at least in the other room. You can always check your phone after 30 minutes has passed.

What will you do to the notifications that your mind throws at you? Ask yourself, is it important? If the answer is YES, write it down in a notebook to work on it later. Re-focus to your activity.

2. Fit your skill and attractiveness of the work in hand – This is based on the level of skill you have for the work in hand and attractiveness of the work-in-hand to you. Please categorize your task in hand to know. The work in hand can be classified as following –

b. High skill – high attractiveness: This only happens when a person is working with a purpose to improve his skill and to change the way the world works for

good at every moment of his life. The skill wants to improve every moment due to an intrinsic motivation. The work in hand continuously challenges the motivated person to overcome it. The senses and time sense while working on it vanishes. Legends work in this zone– always and every day of their lives. We also in some part of our life have felt this state of mind.

c. **High skill-** low attractiveness: It's almost always felt to be a boring task. Avoid distractions at any cost and try to finish as fast as possible. That converts a mundane work interesting many a times.

d. **Low skill-** High attractiveness: You need to develop the skill here. It will take time. Develop a detailed plan to acquire the skill. Start executing your plan in fractions daily. Then start taking the challenges involved in the task which seem reasonable. Thus, you can acquire any skill almost at the expert level within atime of three years, if you work two hours daily for it. Attend workshops. Do short-term certificates, read books, and ask for advice from the experts if possible. Stay motivated.

e. **Low skill-** low attractiveness: It is very difficult to focus. You will waste your time by chasing such task. It's a sure way of destroying your career and yourself.

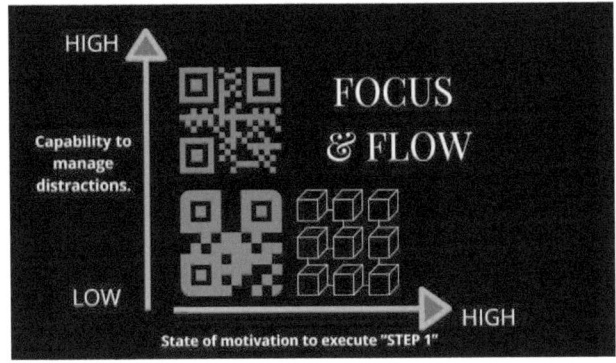

3. Habit of mindfulness breathing– Bring your attention to your breath as your mind starts chasing something else. Slow down your breathing and concentrate on the now.

What to do?

1. Journaling– Note how many times a day you are drifting into unproductive thoughts. Write about them and also about what productive thoughts you should focus instead.

2. Mindful living- Be aware of your unproductive thoughts as you go through your day. Discard these useless thoughts, at will. Fill your mind with productive thoughts that will serve your purpose in life. The ideas that do not provoke any action on your part must also be discarded.

Sense of productivity is required more than we can imagine. In "Step 1" sense and focus are the most important components of productive living. A small percentage change in overall daily productivity can do miracles in the coming years for you, your family, your company and your nation.

Transform With the Muscle of Gratitude

"Gratitude is a vaccine, an antitoxin, and an antiseptic."
~ John Henry Jowett, 1863 – 1923

The past is not in our hands and neither is the future. We can only work in present, by learning from the past and work in a productive way for the future. But our mind wanders a lot to the past as well as future (at-least 46% of the time it wanders). It ruminates and it ruminates mostly about the bad things. So the negative bias increases our state of negative rumination and thus we become less productive.

Our mind is negatively biased, as these negative biases are coming from our evolution; the "evolution of survival" generated these negative biases. Most of this high negativity is not required in today's relatively safe offices and other social environments compared to the jungle where we hunted once upon a time.

A wandering mind is an "unhappy mind." A focused and working mind, which is in the present for the productivity in the future, is the "happiest" mind.

WHAT IS GRATITUDE?

Gratitude is a trait and a state. The state of gratitude results from appreciating a benefit as a positive outcome. Trait gratitude is life-orientation towards noticing and appreciating the little things in life, and other people in our lives. We are happy because we are grateful, and not the other way around.

Gratitude, no matter if it is expressed or received, releases dopamine in the brain. Dopamine is produced in the substantia nigra (where movement and speech are formed) and the ventral tegmental (where reward takes place). Releasing dopamine makes the connection between the behaviour and feeling of goodness. The more a person practices gratitude, the more often dopamine gets released.

Research suggests that gratitude is not a cultural construct; it is embedded in our brain and DNA. Studies have found that chimpanzees are more likely to share food with a chimpanzee that had groomed or helped them in the past.

Cicero, Seneca, Hume, and Adam Smith considered gratitude to be a virtue. Along with them Judaism, Christianity, Islam, Buddhism, and Hinduism all encourage cultivating gratitude as an important moral virtue. The "gratitude to God" is what binds religious people together. This was proved in a study where the brain's response to feelings of gratitude was measured using an fMRI (Functional magnetic resonance imaging). Gratitude increased activity in areas of the brain that deal with morality, reward, and judgment. If gratitude is associated with morality, it supports why philosophical and religious thinkers have used gratitude in the formation and maintenance of their societies.

HOW TO FEEL GRATITUDE?

Here are simple ways to become more grateful:

- The best exercise for gratitude is the daily gratitude journal: Writing things are more powerful than just remembering them. Write on paper, smartphone or computer: "I am grateful for ..." The things you are grateful for are bigger than your problems. Some days you will write without feeling a shred of gratitude but keep practicing, gratitude will come. Do this when you first wake in the morning or late at night before you go to sleep. We all want to be happy and feel good and although it may seem hard to achieve, it is free. The more you feel grateful, the more you'll be happier! Regular gratitude journaling has been shown to result in 5% to 15% increases in optimism and 25% increased sleep quality. A study on gratitude visits showed that participants experienced a 35% reduction in depressive symptoms for several weeks, while those practicing gratitude journaling reported a similar reduction in depressive symptoms for as long as the journaling continued. This is an amazing finding and suggests that gratitude journaling can be an effective supplement to the treatment for depression.

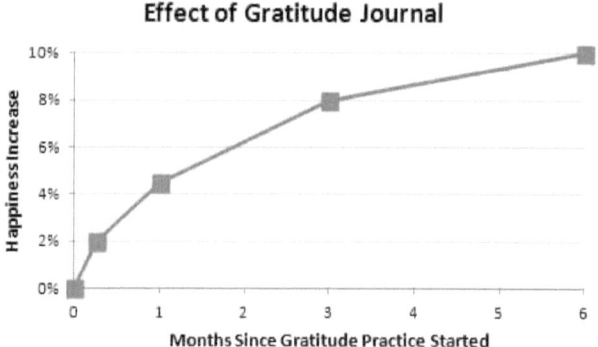

- Gratitude mapping: You place a whiteboard somewhere you can see it every day. On it, you write or draw everything you are grateful for.

- Gratitude jars: When something good happens, you write it down on a piece of paper and put it in a jar. When something bad happens, you read a message from the jar. You pass through bad times remembering the good ones. Remember the bad ones are the indications to learn and improve yourself. Learn from it in detail to upgrade your thinking and ways of doing things. March ahead, and thank that bad event for being your teacher and teaching you a lesson.

- Mindfulness: No matter how much we practice gratitude we are still bound to feel negative emotions like disappointment, guilt, vulnerability, and grief. Happy life means that these are acknowledged and accepted. Mindfulness helps us react to our misfortunes with grace, acceptance, and meditation. Gratitude reduces toxic aggression, frustration, and regret even after receiving negative feedback. Learn from both good and bad. Consider them as your teachers. Thank them for teaching you and move on.

- Prayer: No matter the religion or cultural aspects, just pray to something bigger than you.

- Volunteering: Professor, Martin Seligman, supports in his research *Flourish: A Visionary New Understanding of Happiness and Well-Being*, that volunteering is the single most reliable way to momentarily increase your well-being.

- Practice the Naikan Reflection which is a self-reflection method initially developed in Japan. The process involves reflecting on the following three questions while focusing one's attention on a particular person and time.

1. What did this person give to me? (giving)
2. What did I return to this person? (receiving)
3. What trouble did I cause this person? (hurting)

- Write a letter to someone. When you write about how grateful you are to others it becomes harder for you to think about your negative experiences. You may want to write a letter of gratitude to someone, but you're unsure whether you want that person to read the letter. Actually, it doesn't matter if you send it or not. Simply writing the letter can help you appreciate the people in your life and shift your focus away from negative feelings and thoughts. This is an excellent communication tool for romantic partners.

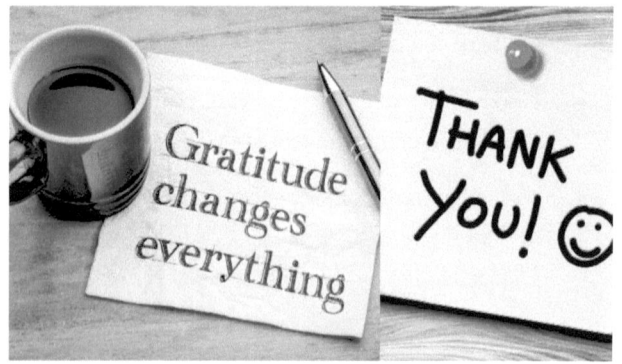

- Use a grateful vocabulary: The words we use build what we feel. In a study of 800 descriptive trait words, "grateful" was rated in the top 4% in terms of likeability. Using words like the great, exceptional, gift-giving increases our state.

STUDIES AND RESEARCH

Gratitude as a "social glue:" There are several studies that link gratitude to prosocial behaviour. These studies show that the more grateful the person is the more helpful and generous he/she are. The studies over gratitude found these psychological characteristics of grateful people:

- They are more agreeable, more open, and less neurotic. Gratitude is inversely connected to depression, and positively to life satisfaction.
- People who express their gratitude for each other tend to be more willing to forgive others and be less narcissistic.
- People who focus on gratitude are more optimistic in general. This makes them more likely to act in ways that support a healthy lifestyle.
- People who write and deliver a letter to someone, for whom they are grateful, tend to have a higher level of happiness and satisfaction.
- In a study by McCraty and colleagues (1998), 45 adults were taught to "cultivate appreciation and other positive emotions." There was a 23% reduction in the stress hormone, cortisol, after the intervention period.

Studies suggest that gratitude may be associated with other virtues, like:

- Patience: One study asked participants to make a series of choices between receiving smaller amounts of cash immediately and larger amounts from six months later. Participants with higher trait gratitude were more likely to wait and take the larger amounts, suggesting that gratitude may reduce impatience.

- Humility: One study found that people who wrote letters expressing gratitude to a significant person in their life displayed more humility than those who completed a different activity that didn't foster gratitude. In the same study, participants were instructed to keep a diary for two weeks. They found that "humility and gratitude mutually predicted one another."

- Wisdom: A study found that people who were considered wise by others expressed more feelings of gratitude than people who weren't singled out by others for their wisdom.

A study by Wong and Brown (2017) wanted to find out how gratitude affects us mentally and physically. Students were placed into three groups:

1. Group one wrote a letter of gratitude to another person every week for three weeks

2. Group two wrote about their thoughts and feelings about negative experiences.

3. Group three didn't write anything.

All three groups received counselling services. Group one reported "significantly better mental health four and 12 weeks" after the intervention ended. Also, a combined gratitude practice/ counselling approach is more beneficial than counselling alone.

HOW GRATITUDE INFLUENCES PHYSICAL HEALTH?

The influence of gratitude on health remains a somewhat understudied area. Still, some promising studies do exist:

- According to a 2004 research, from Harvard Medical School and Massachusetts General Hospital, acute coronary syndrome patients experienced greater improvements in health-related quality of life and greater reductions in depression and anxiety when they approached recovery with gratitude and optimism.

- A study from 2003, and a newer one from 2020, showed that that regularly practicing gratitude can help ease symptoms of anxiety and depression.

- A 2009 study found that people who practiced grateful thoughts before bed fell asleep faster, slept longer, and felt less tired during the day. This may be because practicing gratitude can help calm you down and even lower your heart rate.

- A 2017 study found that people who reported feeling more grateful in their lives had lower blood levels of haemoglobin A1c (HbA1c), an important measure of how well your blood sugar is controlled.

- Gratitude increases the likelihood of physical activity. Exercise provides a huge benefit to both physical and psychological health. In an 11-week study of 96 Americans, those who kept a weekly gratitude journal spent an extra 40 minutes exercising than the control group.

- Individuals with chronic illnesses, due to the long-term and often the pain, develop depression. In one study, investigating these groups, it was determined that those who rated higher on a gratitude questionnaire experienced less depression and less physical pain. Research, as limited as it is, suggests a correlation between gratitude and improved outcomes in cardiac patients.

- According to a 2012 study published in *Personality and Individual Differences*, grateful people experience fewer aches and pains and report feeling healthier than other people. Not surprisingly, grateful people are also more likely to take care of their health. They exercise more often and are more likely to attend regular check-ups, which is likely to contribute to further longevity.

Benefits at a Glance

Results1	Study	Date
Keeping a gratitude journal caused participants to report 16% fewer physical symptoms, 19% more time spent exercising, 10% less physical pain, 8% more sleep, and 25% increased sleep quality	Counting Blessings Versus Burdens	2003
The emotions of appreciation and gratitude shown to **induce the relaxation response.**	The Grateful Heart	2004
A gratitude visit **reduced depressive symptoms by 35%** for several weeks. a gratitude journal lowered depressive symptoms by 30%+ for as long as the practice was continued.	Positive Psychology Progress	2005
Patients with hypertension were instructed to count their blessings once a week. There was a **significant decrease in their systolic blood pressure.**	Gratitude: Effects on Perspectives and Blood Pressure	2007
Gratitude correlated with **improved sleep quality** ($r = 29$), **less time required to fall asleep** ($r = 20$), and **increased sleep duration** ($r = 14$).	Gratitude Influences Sleep Through the Mechanism of Pre-Sleep Cognitions	2009
Levels of gratitude significantly correlated with **vitality and energy**	Multiple Studies	Many

HOW DOES GRATITUDE INFLUENCE MENTAL HEALTH?

- Gratitude reduces envy, resentment, frustration, and regret. Robert Emmons, a leading gratitude researcher, has conducted multiple studies on the link between gratitude and well-being. His research confirms that gratitude effectively increases happiness and reduces depression.

- Gratitude enhances empathy and reduces aggression. Grateful people are more likely to behave in a prosocial manner, even when others behave less kindly, according to a 2012 study by the University of Kentucky. Study participants who ranked higher on gratitude scales were less likely to retaliate against others, even when given negative feedback. They experienced more sensitivity and empathy towards other people and a decreased desire to seek revenge.

- Gratitude increases mental strength. Gratitude reduces not only stress but also plays a major role in overcoming trauma. A 2006 study found that Vietnam War veterans with higher levels of gratitude experienced lower rates of PTSD. A 2003 study found that gratitude was a major contributor to resilience following the terrorist attacks on September 11.

- Being an optimistic person can have plenty of health benefits, including healthy aging, according to a 2019 study. If you're not naturally optimistic, gratitude practice can help you cultivate an optimistic outlook, as suggested by a 2018 study.

- In a 2003 study, it took just 10 weeks of regular gratitude practice for participants to feel more optimistic and positive about their present lives and the future.

- Gratitude not only improves your physical and mental well-being but it may also improve your relationships. Gratitude plays a key role in forming relationships, as well as in strengthening existing ones. When it comes to romantic relationships, gratitude can help partners feel more satisfied with each other. A study in 2010 showed that partners who demonstrated gratitude towards one another reported increased relationship satisfaction and improved happiness in the following days.

Gratitude also affects our work. Here are some incredible statistics about the influence of gratitude at the workplace:

- 70% of employees would feel better about themselves if their bosses were more grateful, and 81% would work harder.

- Employees who experience more gratitude at work report fewer depressive symptoms and stress.

- 95% of employees agree that a grateful boss is more likely to be successful.

- Lack of gratitude is a major factor in driving job dissatisfaction, turnover, absenteeism, and burnout.

- 53% of employees would stay at their company longer if they felt more appreciation from their boss.

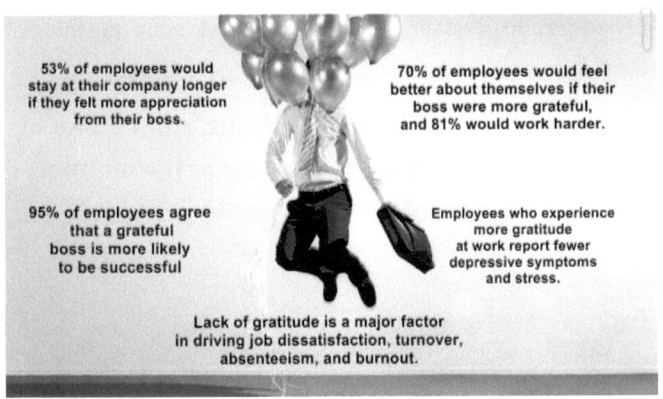

"Gratitude turns what we have into enough, and more. It turns denial into acceptance, chaos into order, confusion into clarity . . . it makes sense of our past, brings peace for today, and creates a vision for tomorrow." - Beattie Melody

When you practice gratitude the world is no longer a battle-field, but a park. The experience of gratitude encourages us to appreciate what is good in our lives and compels us to pay this goodness forward. People with more grateful dispositions report about being happier and more satisfied with their lives.

Positive psychology has been linked with superior cardiovascular health. Positive psychology defines "gratitude" in a way where scientists can measure its effects, and thus argue that gratitude is more than feeling thankful. It is a deeper appreciation that produces longer-lasting positivity.

Gratitude also functions as the social glue that nurtures the formation of new friendships, enriches our existing relationships, and underlies the very foundation of human society. Life satisfaction and gratitude are connected. They include better mental and physical health, more pro-social behaviour, high-quality relationships, and more meaningful lives. Life satisfaction is a key predictor of well-being.

> **"Got no checkbooks, got no banks, still I'd like to express my thanks. I got the sun in the morning and the moon at night."**
>
> *-Irving Berlin*

Expression of gratitude –

1. Mindfulness practices of gratitude. Practice expanding the light of love and gratitude.
2. Directly to the people with proper attention.
3. Express gratitude with a letter by meeting a person.
4. Writing E-mail or letter of gratitude.

The more we practice gratitude – more the muscle of gratitude develops. The more it develops the happier we become in the present. We become more focused. The power of transformation of emotions increases. Give thanks to the "GOOD," give thanks to the "BAD" for teaching you lessons. And you will find soon that those apparent good and bad events or persons actually taught you very important lessons of life. You actually needed those lessons. We rise to our challenges with more positive energy if we have a sense of gratitude by our side; thus we become more productive and successful in life.

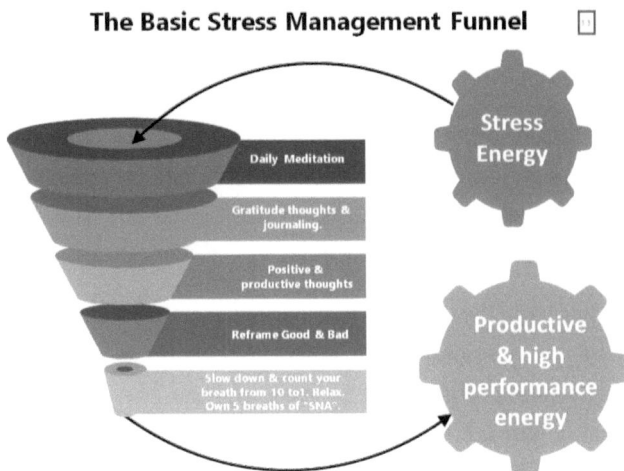

Figure 12: Showing basic stress management funnel.

Minimalism

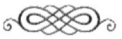

We human beings love varieties. As we built our civilization, we brought a significant number of types into everything. We went on fighting the monotonous offerings of our nature and created many creative distractions for ourselves.

In the last 20 years, we have created more such distractions than the previous 2000 years. A significant number of products and choices are pouring into our lives. These are coming through shopping malls, e-commerce websites, and social media, almost from every direction. Along with this, a significant amount of information about these products and their benefits also pouring into our minds. Our mind is designed to track these varieties closely, and if possible enjoy; we would like to enjoy them as the first-person to do so.

Problems of so many choices and so much information -

1. **Hedonic adaptation-** Human beings have a psychological factor responsible for our continuous progression in our evolution and civilization. The factor is "we are never happy for what we already have." We become adapted to new things or new situations within a few months, new relationships within a few years, etc. This phenomenon is known as "hedonic adaptation." The more we are exposed to modern things, what we can buy or consume daily, the more hedonically we will be adapted to the things that we already have.

2. Now the next problem is that the more we hedonically get adapted to newer things by newer varieties daily, the more we lack happiness and motivation in the NOW. We can become happy now and work now. We cannot get a thing and then become satisfied – if we use to get something only without being HAPPY now, we become stressed. We get things which are supposed to make us happy, but now, even after possessing it, we don't reach that level of happiness or even satisfaction. This lack of excitement, in turn, leads us towards stress. Happiness is a muscle that we lose. On top of that, when you will get those new things, you will soon be adapted to your new status or things. This continues. Thus, you will remain unhappy throughout your life.

3. We want to buy new things daily that we may not even use in the future. We purchase new houses, new cars, new clothes, and so on. To purchase these things, we need to earn more. Our life becomes busier. But for what? Maybe it is for that mindless buying which is either influenced by media or by friends and society. We have become so busy and we are always working.

We are busy multi-tasking. We can focus and perform one activity only at any point in time. We have only one powerful processor which can perform a series of tasks. But doing multiple tasks, simultaneously and perfectly, is a myth.

Always-ON mobile notifications are nothing short of a curse. The same is true for browsing e-commerce and social medial for hours.

These produce a sense of global level comparison, envy and produce rapid hedonic adaptation in those that we already have. Thus it makes us unhappy and more stressed.

1. We become so busy that we overlook our nutrition, exercise and even sleep. We become a compromise; thus we suffer health-related problems. Consumption also increases our carbon footprint as an individual, and therefore it's a burden on earth and our environment.

2. The busy person never has time to look back into his mind. He becomes less and less self-aware and mindful about himself and his surroundings. Here come the issues with our relationships with our families and friends. The lesser the time, focus and energy we spend on these, which we consider that we already have, the more these relationships decay. We lose essential social and also family support sometimes.

3. Now, let's point the discussion into those things that we own. It occupies both our inner (mental) and outer space (house). Our outer space is occupied by so many unnecessary things that "managing them" becomes a big task. We use only 30% of our collections, 80% of the time, approximately. Rest are just occupying spaces. It is neither pleasant visually nor mentally.

   We are also busy inside; your mind is running after money as we are somehow misguided by the fact that earning money would be the solution to our peace of mind and happiness. Science has proven that earning money, more than what we need to live a meaningful life, does not make us happy. What would be a meaningful life? Fulfilling basic needs (house, clothes, food, and education) and then balancing our relationships and passions of our life. Owning things never makes us happy for long. That will remain the truth no matter how hard we try to compensate the required balance by only earning money.

4. More stress and less productivity- When a person is only chasing after money and buying things, it doesn't produce any satisfaction. He runs after money and power more. But as I already told you, owning things and chasing after money for our basic needs to be fulfilled does not significantly improve life satisfaction.

5. Our lifetime is limited. Say, we survive for 70 years; in the first ten years, we spend learning fundamental rules about the world. So what remains is 60 years, out of which we one-third of the time we spend sleeping and around 20% of the time we spend on toilets, eating things, making journeys, etc. The remaining 45% of the time, that means we have around 11 hours in our hands daily, is spent doing something productive. Sharp focus is not possible for more than 6 hours a day. Science says 46% of the time our mind wanders so, mindful living is possible only 6 hours a day. Therefore, on an average, we can live 15 years mindfully.

That is the time that we productively use to educate ourselves, do productive work, take part in building relationships, mindfully, and building a meaningful life around our passion and purpose.

Time is short.

Using this precious energy of focus to store money and things, and then spending time managing those purposeless things are not meaningful. It does not produce that deep sense of satisfaction that we are running after.

Reframe concept of minimalism –

- ❖ Minimalism means depriving ourselves– NO. Rather minimalism means a deep sense of satisfaction with fewer things because you cannot enjoy so many things and also have your peace of mind.

- ❖ Minimalism means poor men's life– NO. Minimalism means leading life by your terms. Keeping things that you need, doing useful things, thinking productive thoughts, earning money that is useful and building relationships not in terms of quantity but with the highest quality.

- ❖ Minimalism means earning less money– NO. Minimalism means more productivity. A productive person will eventually make more money, no matter what. But earning money will impose much lesser stress on him, and he does not do things just because he can. He would be doing something that has a personalized purpose and meaning attached to it.

Bring the Pareto principle in your life –

"You use only 20% of your things daily for your 80% activities," "Your 20% thoughts and words can be 80% effective if chosen mindfully," "Your 20% actions will bring 80% of your desired effects mostly" and so on. De-clutter and organize your life around the Pareto principle. Life will be less stressful.

Minimalism decision matrix

Depending on two factors, we can build a decision-making matrix as follows–

Factor A: Versatility in choice of things, and

Factor B: Productivity of a person.

If a person has excellent versatility in choice and spends hours maintaining those, but is a highly productive fellow (a professional) then his life is full of stress. Life is a meaningless journey for him without any sense of satisfaction.

In those people who do not have a productive mind too, factor A is very high. They spend life chasing ghosts. They imitate what others are doing. They want to satisfy their society by showing things. And will thus never able to benefit themselves.

Where A & B both are low– They are peaceful. But the productivity for their progress is also missing. Here, life satisfaction is also less as the person is not building a life around his purpose and passion.

Where Factor A is low with a very high sense of productivity– the person is a true minimalist.

A minimalist saves his most precious resources to save his time. And thus, he spends his "focus" and "energy" on doing great and productive things. He designs his life around his meaning of life, his passion, and his purpose. He lives his life with a more profound sense of satisfaction, with fewer things and within his own terms. Mastering the power of minimalism is your life; be the minimalist.

Managing things with minimalism

Categorize your products with two factors –

Factor A- Usage frequency – High/ Low,

Factor B– Productive purpose for NOW & FUTURE.

1. You will probably find approximately 30% things that you own, having both the factors high. Keep those things right in front of you to be readily available for use. Arrange for the betterment and maintenance of those products.

2. Approximately 40% of things in your house have both the factors low– please dispose of them, at least physically. You will free lots of space in your home. You can always take pictures of those to preserve the memory of the things. You can write a journal about those.

3. Approximately 10% of items will be there, which has very high productivity– but you are not using them. Take care of those items in freed up spaces, which are

mostly accessible; keep them in a place where your eyes go at least twice a day.

4. And the last categories of items (around 20%) are the ones you are frequently using, but productivity is not there. They are not adding any value to your life. It is better to keep them away from your sight and your reach. Thenslowly discard them, as well.

Be mindful while using the things that add value to your life. Enjoy the satisfaction of a lesser but productive choice of items. It's a practice, which may take some time and patience. But minimalism is worth practicing.

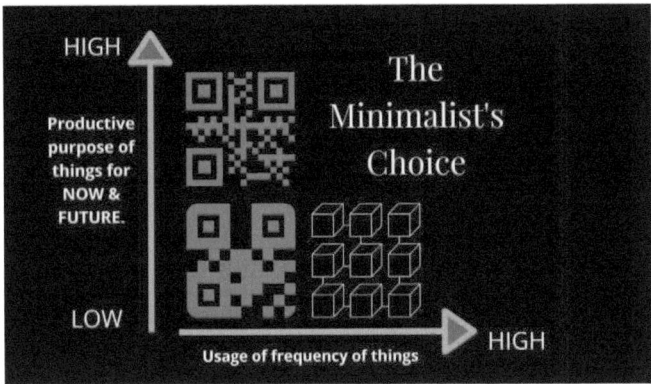

The same categories are valid for each part of our life, our relationships, thoughts, and activities. You can always bring the principles of minimalism in many areas of your life. You will find more peace of mind, more satisfaction, and more time for yourself. I wish you all best of luck.

Own the power of "Impermanence" & "Time."

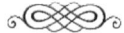

"Right now, the new is you,

but someday not too long from now,

you will gradually become the old and be cleared away.

Sorry to be so dramatic, but it is quite true."

-Steve Jobs

Everything that is around you, including yourself, will not be there forever. The toys that you own as a baby and as an adult (cars, clothes, house and so many other things) will become obsolete and vanish one day. You may think that this is a philosophy. No, it is not. What can be more apparent and real than death itself? The ultimate outcome of life lies in degeneration and death.

Begin your day from the day you would have died. You are lying in a bed, and people are talking about your contribution to earth as a father, as a friend, as a husband, as a professional, or as an innovator. In what way do you want people to remember you? Own that way to be the course of your life. Own that as your purpose of living a meaningful life. Own the power of death to pump the fuel of inspiration into your life.

Everything that we create is earth to the earth's supply chain. Everything that we are on earth is, again, earth to the earth's supply chain. We own some of those items in between when we live and we feel proud or deprived or sad or happy with those things. The supply chain happens, outside, in the world. The reactions occur inside our minds. Own the power of impermanence to know that these are a part of the drama, and when these dramas will end, nothing will remain. In that way, these things will have less power in your mind.

You may praise good things. But do not make them your "needs," and do not make those things your "life." Experience things but do not own them as your "life."

All we have is the "time" which we cannot buy. We can't work in the past. We can't work in the future. We can only work in the present. We can only live in the present; the "present" is all we have. We have had the past experiences and we can try to have the future goals. But we neither can live nor work in the past or in the future. So we must savour every moment as it passes by.

Death is inevitable; so enjoy the togetherness, enjoy the conflicts, the ups and downs, the bad times and the good times. Be the "non-judgmental awareness."

Impermanence propels us in the direction of our passion and purpose. It provides us with the sense to take positive and productive actions in life. It inspires us to take the challenges in life and then take the necessary steps to design life in a way that makes those challenges useless.

The only thing we have is the journey itself. Enjoy the journey. Be happy now. Be the observer and perform your role in the drama as things happen. Let yourself know when this drama will end, nothing will remain except your deeds and the memories of how you did those. Own this power of impermanence to sail through the ups and downs in life. As the people pass you by and conclude their own dramas, celebrate their memories, celebrate those moments you spend together, celebrate life at your best. The mourning is for you only; it does not involve those who have already become your past. The past has already happened and you can't do anything about it.

Whenever things feel gloomy, do not mourn; bring the power of impermanence back into your thoughts and control the situation. Draw inspiration from impermanence, observe the situations as they are, and do not judge. When the right time comes, be sure to jump into the action.

Own the power of impermanence to live life at its fullest. Live every moment with the joy of impermanence.

References:

1. The brain on silent: mind wandering, mindful awareness, and states of mental tranquility David R. Vago1 and Fadel Zeidan2 1Functional Neuroimaging Laboratory, Brigham & Women's Hospital and Department of Psychiatry, Harvard Medical School, Boston, Massachusetts 2 Department of Neurobiology and Anatomy, Wake Forest School of Medicine, Winston-Salem, North Carolina

2. Effects of Mindfulness on Psychological Health: A Review of Empirical Studies Shian-Ling Keng, Moria J. Smoski, and Clive J. Robins Department of Psychology and Neuroscience, Duke University,

Durham, NC 27708 Department of Psychiatry and Behavioral Sciences, Duke University Medical Center, Durham, NC 27710 Correspondence concerning this paper should be addressed to Shian-Ling Keng, Box 3026, Duke University Medical Center, Durham, NC 27710. slk18@duke.edu, Phone: (1) 919-309-6226, Fax: (1) 919-684-6770

3. Mindfulness, psychological well-being and psychological distress in adolescents: Assessing the mediating variables and mechanisms of autonomy and self-regulation Moslem Partoa *, Mohammad Ali Besharatb a Department of counseling and Psychology, Research Institute for Education, P. O. Box 14169-35671, Tehran, Iran b Department of Psychology, University of Tehran, P. O. Box 14155-6456, Tehran, Iran

4. Gratitude and Well Being The Benefits of Appreciation Randy A. Sansone, MD and Lori A. Sansone, MD Randy A. Sansone, Dr. R. Sansone is a professor in the Departments of Psychiatry and Internal Medicine at Wright State University School of Medicine in Dayton, Ohio, and Director of Psychiatry Education at Kettering Medical Center in Kettering, Ohio;

5. The impact of mindfulness on wellbeing and performance in the workplace: An inclusive systematic review of the empirical literature. Authors Tim Lomas1†, Juan Carlos Medina2 , Itai Ivtzan1 , Silke Rupprecht3 , Rona Hart1, Francisco Eiroa-

Orosa1 1 School of Psychology, University of East London, Arthur Edwards Building, Water Lane, London, E15 4LZ, United Kingdom 2 Faculty of Psychology, University of Barcelona, Passeig de la Vall d'Hebron, 08035 Barcelona, Spain 3 Leuphana University, Scharnhorststraße 1, 21335 Lüneburg, Germany

6. Mindfulness and Well-Being By Shawn R. Englund-Helmeke Research Chair: Sarah Ferguson, MA, MSW, Ph.D. Committee Members: Carey Winkler, MSW, LICSW; Leslie Colerin, MSW Clinical Research Paper Presented to the Faculty of the School of Social Work St. Catherine University and the University of St. Thomas St. Paul, Minnesota

7. Promoting Psychological Well-Being Through an Evidence-Based Mindfulness Training Program Yi-Yuan Tang1 *, Rongxiang Tang2 and James J. Gross 3 1Department of Psychological Sciences, Texas Tech University, Lubbock, TX, United States, 2Department of Psychological and Brain Sciences, Washington University in St. Louis, St. Louis, MO, United States, 3Department of Psychology, Stanford University, Stanford, CA, United States

8. Chadwick P, Hember M, Symes J, Peters E, Kuipers E, Dagnan D. Responding mindfully to unpleasant thoughts and images: Reliability and validity of the Southampton Mindfulness

Questionnaire (SMQ) British Journal of Clinical Psychology. 2008;47:451–455. [PubMed]
[Google Scholar]

Chadwick P, Taylor KN, Abba N. Mindfulness groups for people with psychosis. Behavioural and Cognitive Psychotherapy. 2005;33:351–359. [Google Scholar]

9. Chambers R, Gullone E, Allen NB. Mindful emotion regulation: An integrative review. Clinical Psychology Review. 2009;29:560–572. [PubMed] [Google Scholar]

10. Chambers R, Lo BCY, Allen NB. The impact of intensive mindfulness training on attentional control, cognitive style, and affect. Cognitive Therapy and Research. 2008;32:303–322.[Google Scholar]

11. Chiesa A, Serretti A. Mindfulness based cognitive therapy for psychiatric disorders: A systematic review and meta-analysis. Psychiatry Research 2010 in press. [PubMed] [Google Scholar]

12. Coelho HF, Canter PH, Ernst E. Mindfulness-based cognitive therapy: Evaluating current evidence and informing future research. Journal of Consulting and Clinical Psychology. 2007;75:1000–1005. [PubMed] [Google Scholar]

13. Cordon SL, Brown KW, Gibson PR. The role of mindfulness-based stress reduction on perceived stress: Preliminary evidence for the moderating role of attachment style. Journal of Cognitive

Psychotherapy: An International Quarterly. 2009;23:258–268. [Google Scholar] Crane C, Barnhofer T, Duggan D, Hepburn S, Fennell MV, Williams JMG. Mindfulness-based cognitive therapy and self-discrepancy in recovered depressed patients with a history of depression and suicidality. Cognitive Therapy & Research. 2008;32:775–787. [Google Scholar]

14. Craigie MA, Rees CS, Marsh A, Nathan P. Mindfulness-based cognitive therapy for generalized anxiety disorder: A preliminary evaluation. Behavioural and Cognitive Psychotherapy.

2008;36:553–568. [Google Scholar]

15. Creswell JD, Way BM, Eisenberger NI, Lieberman MD. Neural correlates of dispositional mindfulness during affect labeling. Psychosomatic Medicine. 2007;69:560–565. [PubMed] [Google Scholar]

16. Davidson R. Well-being and affective style: neural substrates and biobehavioral correlates.

Philosophical Transactions of the Royal Society. 2004;359:1395–1411. [PMC free article] [PubMed] [Google Scholar]

17. Davidson RJ. Emotion and affective style: hemispheric substrates. Psychological Science.

1992;3:39–43. [Google Scholar]

18. Davidson RJ, Kabat-Zinn J, Schumacher J, Rosenkranz M, Muller D, Santorelli SF, Sheridan JF.

Alterations in brain and immune function produced by mindfulness meditation. Psychosomatic Medicine. 2003;65:564–570. [PubMed] [Google Scholar]

19. Davis KM, Lau MA, Cairns DR. Development and preliminary validation of a trait version of the Toronto Mindfulness Scale. Journal of Cognitive Psychotherapy: An International Qaurterly.

2009;23:185–197. [Google Scholar]

20. Dekeyser M, Raes F, Leijssen M, Leysen S, Dewulf D. Mindfulness skills and interpersonal behaviour. Personality and Individual Differences. 2008;44:1235–1245. [Google Scholar]

21. Ehring T, Watkins E. Repetitive negative thinking as a transdiagnostic process. International Journal of Cognitive Therapy. 2008;1:192–205. [Google Scholar]

22. Eifert GH, Heffner M. The effects of acceptance versus control contexts on avoidance of panicrelated symptoms. Journal of Behavior Therapy and Experimental Psychiatry. 2003; 34:293–312.[PubMed] [Google Scholar]

23. Epstein-Lubow G, McBee L, Darling E, Armey M, Miller I. A pilot investigation of mindfulness-based stress reduction for caregivers of frail elderly. Mindfulness in press.[Google Scholar]

24. Froh JJ, Kashdan TB, Ozimkowski KM, Miller N. Who benefits the most from a gratitude intervention in children and adolescents? Examining positive affect as a moderator. J Posit Psychol.2009;4:408–422. [Google Scholar]

25. Polak EL, McCullough ME. Is gratitude an alternative to materialism? J Happiness Stud. 2006;7:343–360. [Google Scholar]

26. Kashdan TB, Uswatte G, Julian T. Gratitude and hedonic and eudaimonic well-being in Vietnam war veterans. Behav Res Ther. 2006;44:177–199. [PubMed] [Google Scholar]

27. Gurel Kirgiz O. Effects of gratitude on subjective well-being, self-construal, and memory. Diss Abstr Int. 2008;68:4825B. [Google Scholar]

28. Henrie P. The effects of gratitude on divorce adjustment and well-being of middle-aged divorced women. Diss Abstr Int. 2007;67:6096B. [Google Scholar]

29. Mallen Ozimkowski K. The gratitude visit in children and adolescents: an investigation of gratitude and subjective well-being. Diss Abstr Int. 2008;69:686B. [Google Scholar]

30. Emmons RA, McCullough ME, Tsang J-A. The assessment of gratitude. In: Lopez SJ, Snyder CR,editors. Positive Psychological Assessment: A Handbook of Models and Measures. Washington, DC:American Psychological Association; 2003. pp. 327–341. [Google Scholar]

31. McCullough ME, Emmons RA. Tsang J-A. The grateful disposition: a conceptual and empirical topography. J Pers Soc Psychol. 2002;82:112–127. [PubMed] [Google Scholar]

32. Watkins PC, Woodward K, Stone T, Kolts RL. Gratitude and happiness: development of a measure of gratitude and relationships with subjective well-being. Soc Behav Pers. 2003;31:431–452. [Google Scholar]

33. Bono G, McCullough ME. Positive responses to benefit and harm: bringing forgiveness and gratitude into cognitive therapy. J Cognit Psychother. 2006;20:147–158. [Google Scholar]

www.ingramcontent.com/pod-product-compliance
Ingram Content Group UK Ltd.
Pitfield, Milton Keynes, MK11 3LW, UK
UKHW042001230426
12048UKWH00009B/477

9 789354 275456